# Your Child's Hearing Loss:

## A Guide for Parents

*Second Edition*

# Your Child's Hearing Loss:

## A Guide for Parents

*Second Edition*

**Debby Waldman**
**Jackson Roush**

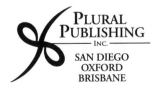

PLURAL
PUBLISHING
— INC. —
SAN DIEGO
OXFORD
BRISBANE

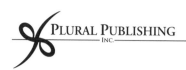

5521 Ruffin Road
San Diego, CA 92123

e-mail: info@pluralpublishing.com
Web site: http://www.pluralpublishing.com

49 Bath Street
Abingdon, Oxfordshire OX14 1EA
United Kingdom

**FSC**
**Mixed Sources**
Product group from well-managed
forests and other controlled sources

Cert no. SW-COC-002283
www.fsc.org
© 1996 Forest Stewardship Council

Typeset in 11/13 Garamond by Flanagan's Publishing Services, Inc.
Printed in the United States of America by McNaughton and Gunn, Inc.
Second printing, March 2010

**Library of Congress Cataloging-in-Publication Data:**

Waldman, Debby.
    Your child's hearing loss : a guide for parents / Debby Waldman and Jackson
Roush. — 2nd ed.
        p. cm.
    Includes bibliographical references and index.
    ISBN-13: 978-1-59756-321-5 (alk. paper)
    ISBN-10: 1-59756-321-8 (alk. paper)
    1. Deafness in children—Popular works. 2. Hearing disorders in children—
Popular works.   I. Roush, Jackson. II. Title.
    RF291.5.C45W355 2009
    618.92'0978—dc22
                                                                        2009024122

# Contents

# Foreword

When I began my career at the Hearing and Speech Clinic in Halifax, Nova Scotia, in 1972, I quickly learned that I preferred working with young children and their families and, in time, I became the pediatric audiologist at this center. Unlike the adults who often chose not to use hearing aids, the hard-of-hearing children and their families with whom I worked were positive and optimistic about hearing instrument technology, such as it was in those years.

Relative to the knowledge and vast array of instrument technology we have today, we had very little to work with in the early 1970s; there were no electrophysiological systems to test the hearing of young infants, no devices to measure the performance of hearing aids, and no systematic way to prescribe hearing aids for children.

Our limitations became especially apparent in the mid-1970s, when a major rubella epidemic broke out in the Canadian Maritime provinces. At that time, the Nova Scotia Hearing and Speech Clinic provided audiology services for three provinces: Nova Scotia, New Brunswick, and Prince Edward Island. Within a month or two of the epidemic, close to 40 babies were referred to our clinic. To this date, I remember the names of many of those babies and the faces of those young mothers and fathers. Because our knowledge of pediatric hearing loss was limited, there was a lot of "guesstimating" but mostly there was a lot of hoping. The young parents kept bringing their babies back and in the process, together, we all learned a great deal.

I made a few observations during this experience. First, I observed that when I was lucky and somehow provided the baby with "appropriate" hearing aids, for which there were only very crude criteria, things began to happen. Most but not all of the babies seemed to be hearing. In fact, some seemed to be hearing very well. Through these experiences, I came to understand how powerful and helpful this work could be.

I also observed that the progress these babies made did not seem to depend entirely on the degree of their hearing loss or the appropriateness of the hearing aid fitting. Certainly, there were babies who appeared to derive little or no benefit from the hearing aids. A number of them had profound hearing losses and, unfortunately, it would be some 15 or more years before cochlear implants would become available for young children. We worked with families to help them to choose the communication option that was best for them and their children.

At the same time, though, I saw that there were some babies with quite severe hearing losses who were making remarkable progress with amplification. In time I concluded that one of the most important factors appeared to be the extent to which the parents (and in many cases, the grandparents) were engaged in the process. Some parents came to our sessions with a seemingly endless list of questions and important observations about their child. In contrast, other parents spent the first year or more flying to Montreal, Toronto, and the United States to get second, third, and fourth opinions about their child's hearing. There was something very important and interesting going on here—something worth learning more about. If we could understand this process better from the parents' perspective, we might then design our services to be more helpful to them.

In 1976 I decided to take my clinical experience and my many questions back to school. At the University of Connecticut, working with pediatric audiology pioneer Dr. Mark Ross, I learned more about the process of hearing aid fitting in preverbal children. I also studied counseling with Dr. Thomas Giolas, who was one of the very few audiologists to recognize the enormous importance of the counseling process in our work with clients and their families.

Since then, my research program has focused on developing a pediatric hearing instrument selection and fitting method so that audiologists and families have a scientific approach to hearing instrument fitting that I did not have in 1972. Along the way, I have learned a great deal from many children, parents, and grandparents. I thank them deeply for this. My life has been enriched greatly through these experiences and, hopefully, I have been of some help to them.

The book Debby Waldman has written with Jack Roush is a great gift to us all. It is a book beautifully written for parents. With great skill, these authors provide the reader with important technical details about hearing loss in children, interwoven with powerful stories from the heart. I only wish that I had had a book like this to read when I began my career. Although the book has been written for parents, it is my fervent hope that it will also be read by audiologists, physicians, early interventionists, speech-language pathologists, educators, and the many students who want to be helpful to children with hearing loss and their families. Thank you, Debby and Jack, for this precious gift.

Richard Seewald, PhD
Distinguished University Professor
   and Canada Research Chair in
   Childhood Hearing
The University of Western Ontario
London, Ontario, Canada

# Preface

When my first child, Elizabeth, was diagnosed with a permanent hearing loss 2 weeks after her third birthday, I was shattered. Although her dad and I had suspected something was wrong with her hearing, neither of us was remotely prepared for the news that she would have to wear hearing aids, we would probably never know what caused the loss, and no operation could fix her ears.

"I'm a surgeon," the pediatric ear, nose, and throat specialist we were sent to after her diagnosis told us. "If I could operate, I would."

Instead of the hospital, we headed to a "dispensing" clinic about 10 minutes from our house, where an audiologist injected blobs of blue putty-like silicone into Elizabeth's ears to make impressions for her first set of earmolds, to go with her first pair of hearing aids.

By this time, my husband, Dave, and I had had a few weeks to adjust to the idea that our daughter really had a hearing problem. We talked out loud about what we'd each realized privately: that Elizabeth could hear when we pressed our lips to one of her ears and spoke into it, but she couldn't hear her 1-year-old brother crying from the other side of the room, and if we called to her from a distance, unless she could see us, she wouldn't know where to find us.

At the clinic that day we collected more pamphlets about hearing loss and hearing aids, which we added to the pile that included brochures from an audiologist in North Dakota (the older sister of one of Elizabeth's babysitters) and from the social worker at the rehabilitation hospital where Elizabeth had undergone the tests that confirmed her hearing loss and where she would eventually attend preschool for hard-of-hearing children.

The brochures were informative, but limited. There was nothing from other parents, nothing to prepare us for how this new reality would affect our daily lives. At the rehab hospital library, I searched the shelves in the Hearing Impairment section and found a variety of books for parents of deaf children, but only one for parents of a child with hearing aids. It was by the mother of a boy who had been diagnosed with a mild-to-moderate hearing loss back in the early 1980s, what I had already come to consider the dark ages of hearing aids for children. The story was interesting, but not exactly relevant to what I was experiencing at the dawn of the 21st century.

In September 1999, about half a year after Elizabeth began wearing hearing aids, she started preschool at the rehab hospital. She had four classmates, all of whom wore hearing aids. I couldn't stop myself from peppering their parents with questions: *How did you find out about your child's loss? How did you deal with it? How often do you change batteries? Have you found a more useful hearing aid cleaning tool than that flimsy little toothpick-with-a-wire contraption that costs two dollars at the clinic and breaks after one use? How often do you have to get new earmolds? Does your child put in his own aids, or do you have to do it? How can you tell the difference between when your child can't hear because the equipment isn't working properly and when she just doesn't want to listen to you?*

The conversations we had were lively and nonstop; we all had questions our audiologists couldn't answer, and our children weren't in elementary school yet. From sessions with the parent liaison at the preschool program, we learned that once elementary school began, we could expect to deal with even more issues.

The germ of the idea for *Your Child's Hearing Loss: A Guide for Parents* was born during the year Elizabeth spent in preschool. Although the professionals who worked with her could and did provide me with technical information about her equipment and educational needs, only other parents helped me understand what I needed to help Elizabeth and the rest of my family on a daily basis.

One of the first things Jack Roush and I did after agreeing to coauthor the first edition of this book was put together a questionnaire for parents of children who were hard of hearing and wore hearing aids, or deaf and used cochlear implants. Our goal was to get enough responses to provide a broad range of experiences. Between the questionnaires and interviews I conducted, including contacts with hard-of-hearing adults and teenagers, we collected more than 40 stories. For this current edition, we interviewed an additional 10 families and followed up on the people we'd interviewed in 2002 and 2003.

No two families had identical experiences, although there were recurring themes. Of those initial 40 families, one third had no trouble getting a diagnosis: their children were tested at birth, through newborn hearing screening programs or as part of testing for a genetic syndrome. Others were tested after an illness, usually meningitis, and so the hearing loss came as no surprise. Another third had no trouble getting a diagnosis after telling their physician they were concerned about their child's behavior. The remaining third, however, had their concerns dismissed by doctors. The implication seemed to be that Mom and Dad were too inexperienced to know the difference between real and imagined problems, and that they were simply worrying too much.

"Doctors said, 'He's a boy, he's a boy, they talk later, blah blah blah,'" recalls Cheri, who began worrying about her middle child, Carter, when he was an infant. Unlike her outgoing and chatty oldest, "Carter just seemed different to me," she says. "He would sit in his car seat and gaze out the window. He wasn't engaged unless he was looking at you. There was a part of me that kept saying oh, no, it couldn't be anything, but I knew something was wrong."

Carter developed the first of many ear infections when he was 2 weeks old. At 9 months, he got his first set of tympanostomy tubes to prevent the accumulation of fluid in his middle ear. The doctor assured Cheri that Carter would be hearing well within a couple of days. A couple of days went by, and Carter still wasn't responding to sounds, so Cheri brought him back to the doctor, who clapped his hands behind the baby's back. When Carter felt the breeze and turned to the source, the doctor said he was fine.

Cheri never went back to that doctor. Instead, she took Carter to an audiologist who was convinced he had some hearing. Still certain there was a problem, Cheri then brought her son to a larger clinic at the University of North Carolina, where he was tested more extensively. That's when she learned her son was profoundly deaf. "I was devastated," she says. "My husband was out of town and I felt like my child had just died. You think, 'Oh my God, he's never going to say my name, he's never going to talk.' The only experience I had with a deaf person was in seventh grade, where I had a phys ed teacher who was deaf. I remember kids making fun of him behind his back, and I thought, 'This is what my son's going to have.' It was really life altering."

Jennifer, too, was an experienced mother when she began wondering if something was wrong with her infant, Danny, though she didn't suspect deafness. An occupational therapist, she wondered if something was wrong with his sensorimotor skills.

"I started asking my pediatrician when Danny was 4 months old if something unusual was going on," she says. "The doctor told me that nothing was wrong and that I, being an occupational therapist, 'knew too much' and was in a sense looking too hard for something to be wrong."

By the time Danny was 9 months old, the pediatrician agreed with Jennifer and ordered blood tests to determine if he had muscle disorders. At 1 year old, Danny was diagnosed with a profound hearing loss.

"It was difficult news to get," Jennifer says. "But having worked with deaf children and children with disabilities, I knew that we—and he—would be okay, and that we would do what was necessary to give him a full life."

When my neighbor, Kathy, read an early draft of this book, one of her first comments was to caution me against scaring parents. Kathy has six daughters. Her youngest, Becky, has a hearing loss similar to Elizabeth's. Her second oldest, Elfi, has spina bifida. One of the first books Kathy read after Elfi was born came with the following caveat: "Marriages rarely last in the case of a child with a disability."

It never occurred to Jack and me to ask parents, in the questionnaire, whether their marriages had survived their child's diagnosis of hearing loss. One parent, herself hard of hearing since birth, said she felt guilty about her child's loss and her husband didn't really understand. But not one said anything about their marriage having broken up as a result. Still, the diagnosis of hearing loss is stressful for any family. Uncertainties and conflicting advice can add to the tension. Mothers often take on the additional burden of "family expert" on matters related to the child's special needs.

A diagnosis of hearing loss can be devastating and most families need time to grieve. Fortunately, much can be done through technology and intervention, and most families eventually cope well. That's not to say that hearing loss is without its recurring frustrations and tensions. I can guarantee it will sometimes eat up more time and energy than you have to spare, that your child will lose or damage his hearing aids, and that a battery will die on the day you've forgotten to put fresh ones in your pocket or purse.

In the grand scheme of things, however, it's something most of us learn to live with. As hard as it is to believe, you may even find things to appreciate about hearing loss. And as Kathy pointed out to me, eventually the child, not you, will take responsibility for the hearing loss.

Elizabeth began taking responsibility for her hearing aids when she was around 7 years old. She could change batteries and she no longer asked me to take out her aids at night or put them in in the morning, though I still cleaned them after she fell asleep. When she was 3 and newly aided, I honestly assumed I'd be doing those tasks until she graduated from high school and left home. But they're her aids, and she wanted to care for them, as she was making increasingly clear.

"You don't own it; the child does," Kathy reminded me. "Essentially, you are teaching the management skills right from the beginning, and she'll teach you."

Kathy was right: by the time Jack and I began revising this book in late 2008, shortly before Elizabeth turned 12, she had assumed responsibility for everything to do with her hearing aids except shopping for batteries and making appointments with the audiologist.

It's my hope and Jack's that this book will help make the process of learning to live with hearing aids and cochlear implants a smoother one for you and your child, and for everyone involved in your child's life.

# Acknowledgments

So many people helped make this book possible and I've done my best to include them here. If I've left anyone out, please accept my apologies.

The first person I must thank is Jack Roush, my writing partner since we began working on the first edition in 2002. His dedication to helping children with hearing loss and their families, combined with his generosity of spirit, made him an ideal coauthor. If it weren't for him, *Your Child's Hearing Loss: A Guide for Parents* would not exist.

Many of the parents and professionals who helped with the first edition, whether by responding to our questionnaires, giving advice, reading drafts, or agreeing to be interviewed, were also involved in this edition. Jack and I are extremely grateful to them all. They include Arthur Ackerhalt, Karen Berger, Joan Black, Dee Ann and Katy Bowen, Sharon and Corey Brady, Cherie Brown, Pamela and Jenny Campbell, Candy Carrier, Cathy Chow, Lori Cochenour, Kim Davis, Rachel de Castro, Sherilynne Di Paolo, Carol Flexer, Trish Freeman, Deborah and Jerry Gideon, Jennifer Glazer, Bruce Goldstein, Melody Harrison, Tannis Howarth, Donna Humphrey, Brad Ingrao, David James, Chantal Kealey, Matthew and Pamela Lang, Paige Lacy, Teresa and Jesse Kazemir, Debbie and Katrina Kuefler, Brenda Mazur, Leigh Reeves, Vicki and Toby Robinson, Pat Roush, Jeanne Safer, Elyse Sass, Diane Schmidt, Stephanie Sjoblad, Pam Sprague, Carren Stika, Arthur and Tracy Tastet, Holly Teagle, Maria and Melissa Tobias, Jennifer Valdis, Kathy Wensel, Karl R. White, Kathryn Wilson, Jill C. Wood, Denise Wray, and Christie Yoshinaga-Itano.

I am especially grateful to Meredith Holcomb, who worked on the original Resources section when she was a graduate student in audiology at the University of North Carolina, and Hannah O'Hare, a current UNC graduate student, who assisted with updates.

I'd like to give a very special thank-you to Richard Seewald, a pioneer in the field of pediatric audiology, for the support he has given to this project since the beginning, and for his beautiful and heartfelt foreword.

Closer to home, I'd like to thank Jan McClelland, Caterina Edwards, and my family: David, Elizabeth, and Noah Wishart, Irlene and Amy Waldman, and Pat and Bill Wishart, for their patience and support.

# Authors' Note

Having a child diagnosed with hearing loss is a new and unfamiliar experience for most families. Our goal for this book is to provide information at a level that is informative to parents without being overly detailed or technical. It is written in first person, but we worked together in an effort to combine technical accuracy with a writing style that would be useful to parents interested in more detail than what is typically offered in booklets and handouts. This book will be of interest primarily to families who choose to communicate with their child using an oral language method in conjunction with hearing aids or a cochlear implant. We respect the right of families to choose a nonoral method such as American Sign Language (ASL) or one of the sign systems that provide a visual representation of English. Information regarding those methods is provided in the Resources. The Resources section also provides sources for additional information on all topics presented in this text, as well as a list of recommended readings and Web sites.

We do not want to mislead parents into thinking that hearing aids or cochlear implants benefit all children equally or that they alone will solve every problem. Some children, especially those with disabilities in addition to hearing loss, may not benefit from either technology. Still, it has been our experience that nearly all children with hearing loss benefit from hearing aids, a cochlear implant or, in some cases, a combination of the two. Our goal is to help parents understand the processes involved in the assessment of hearing, selecting hearing instruments, and various communication options. We also provide information to assist with acquiring and, when necessary, advocating for special services when needed.

Finally, we want to acknowledge that this book is aimed primarily at the practical issues associated with hearing loss in children. You will read some interesting and heartfelt testimonials from parents who share personal aspects of parenting a deaf or hard-of-hearing child, but we make no attempt to present, in depth, the psychoemotional aspects of hearing loss for parents or children. Readers interested in a more detailed exploration of these important issues are referred to several excellent books listed in the Recommended Reading.

The authors welcome comments and suggestions from parents and professionals. Please feel free to contact us via e-mail at debby@debbywaldman.com or jroush@med.unc.edu.

# 1

# IN THE BEGINNING

One of the first things I did after bringing my newborn daughter, Elizabeth, home from the hospital was take her on a tour of the house. Holding her close, I walked from room to room, explaining the origin of each piece of furniture and introducing her to the people in the photos that lined the walls and bookcases.

My husband, Dave, welcomed her home by ringing a bell next to her ear. She didn't seem to notice. "I don't think she can hear," he said.

"You worry too much," I told him. "She's an infant. She can't even turn her head."

When Elizabeth was 14 months old and a proficient walker, Dave wondered why she didn't come to the door to greet him when he arrived home after work.

"She's busy focusing on something else," I said. "She's not like one of the dogs you grew up with—she's not going to fetch your slippers in her teeth and run to the door."

On a business trip when Elizabeth was 17 months old, Dave sat on the plane next to a mother and her 13-month-old daughter. This baby girl could make animal noises. When Dave returned home he talked more about her than he did about his trip.

This time, instead of feeling bad that he was worrying unnecessarily, I was indignant. "The reason Elizabeth can't make animal noises is that I have better things to do all day than sit around and teach her to bark and moo and oink on command."

Thinking back about those moments, I am overwhelmed with two feelings. One is guilt. The other is that there's a lot of merit to the old adage, "Hindsight is 20/20."

It was easy for me to dismiss Dave's concerns: after all, I was with Elizabeth all day, every day, and she didn't seem to have any

1

hearing problems as far as I could tell. When I did worry was when she failed to express any interest in sharing books. During my pregnancy, I'd fantasized about holding my baby on my lap and reading my favorite stories out loud. But as soon as Elizabeth was mobile, she'd crawl off my lap after about the second page and find something that interested her more.

It never occurred to me to call a doctor, much less an audiologist. Instead, I did what came naturally: I asked friends whether their babies liked being read to. Inevitably, when someone told me their child loved books, I felt like a failure. When someone told me their child reacted like Elizabeth, I felt we were both failures.

Elizabeth had no interest in television, either, but far from worrying, I considered that a point of pride, a sign of her discriminating taste: she had more important things to do than spend her time with Barney or Bert and Ernie.

I had no doubt she could hear me and everyone else who talked to her. People often commented on how intently she looked at them when they spoke. "She really makes eye contact!" they would say, and I, the new and naive mommy, proudly agreed. Now, of course, I know she was staring at them not because she had good manners (she was a toddler, for goodness sakes!), but because she was watching their lips.

Perhaps if she'd had trouble talking, I might have taken Dave's concerns more seriously. But she cooed and babbled on schedule, and said her first word, "doggy," when she was 10 months old, pointing to a friend's hyper-bouncy English Springer spaniel.

By the time she was 15 months, her vocabulary was growing steadily. She didn't talk nearly as much as her friend Joseph had when he was her age, but Joseph's toddler vocabulary was more sophisticated than that of many adults I'd encountered. (When he was about 18 months old, he looked up at me one day and said, "How do you like my trousers?") As far as I was concerned, he was the anomaly, not Elizabeth.

The summer that Elizabeth was 2½ and her brother, Noah, 8 months old, Dave and I packed the kids into our brand-new used Toyota Corolla and drove the nearly 3000 miles from Edmonton to Cape Cod, stopping along the way to visit family and friends. Compared to some of our friends' children, Elizabeth seemed quiet—quieter than I remembered her being at home—but Dave and I figured she was shy.

When we got back to Edmonton, though, Elizabeth began having temper tantrums. Up until then, she'd been quite mild-mannered. I'd considered myself blessed to have given birth to a child with such a lovely disposition. Maybe, I thought to myself, she was going through the "terrible twos"?

Joseph was 11 months older than Elizabeth, so one day when we were at his house and Elizabeth was throwing a fit, I asked his mother, "Did Joseph have a lot of tantrums last year at this time?"

She thought for a minute. "No," she said. "He'd pretty well outgrown them by then."

What's wrong with my kid? I wondered, but I had no answer, nor did I have any idea where to look for one.

That fall I signed Elizabeth up for gymnastics, music, and playschool. She missed the first week of playschool because we'd been out of town, but on her first day, she quickly joined a group of girls dressing themselves from a trunk of clothes and pretending to mother a collection of dolls in a playhouse.

After a while, the teacher announced it was time to clean up and get ready for a story. The kids began pitching in to put the toys away. The playhouse girls began tidying up, tossing clothes back into the trunk just outside the door. Elizabeth stayed in the house, oblivious to what was going on around her.

Playschool was held in our neighborhood community hall, an expansive high-ceilinged room with a half dozen oversized windows, shiny linoleum floors, and nothing to absorb the sound of 14 busy preschoolers. But I didn't stop to consider that noise might be the problem. I figured Elizabeth wasn't familiar with the routine, so I stuck my head through the little doorway and called to her, repeating the teacher's words. Then the teacher, who hadn't moved from her spot in the front of the room, made the announcement again. Elizabeth remained in the house, playing. I called to her again. No response.

Eventually Elizabeth left the playhouse. Tired of being alone, she decided to see where her new playmates had gone. The first person to catch her attention was the teacher. Upon seeing the look of impatience and irritation on the teacher's face, which matched the tone of her voice, Elizabeth burst into tears and didn't stop crying for what seemed to me like ages.

I took her aside and comforted her, explaining that the teacher wanted her to clean up, that it was time to listen to a story. By the time I calmed her down, the children were sitting in a circle around the teacher.

Elizabeth took the only available space, directly across the circle from the teacher: she was at 6 o'clock to the teacher's 12. She sat attentively for about 2 minutes. Then she stood up quietly and padded softly away. Nearby was a shelf of toys. She sat quietly in front of it, playing. I didn't urge her back to the circle: she didn't seem to be disturbing anyone, and I didn't want to upset her again. After a minute or two, one of the boys joined her. That's when the teacher told her—and the boy—to come back. I held her on my lap and cuddled her and she remained quiet and well behaved for the rest of the morning.

I took Elizabeth to playschool one more time. This time I stayed for only a short while before kissing her goodbye and telling her I was leaving. In the 5 minutes between when I left the school and arrived home, the teacher called and left a message. "Elizabeth is in tears," she said. "She didn't know where you were. You'd better come back."

So went our first preschool experience. She was too young, I figured. I was neither surprised nor upset. We'd sign her up again in January, after she turned 3. In the meantime, we still had music and gymnastics.

The music teacher held classes in her basement, in a warm and cozy low-ceilinged carpeted room she'd designed especially for that purpose. There were about 10 parents and almost twice as many kids in the room, but it never seemed too noisy, even when the children were hitting drums with sticks, or shaking maracas, or banging on tambourines. Elizabeth seemed to enjoy it immensely; she paid attention and participated along with everyone else.

Gymnastics was another story. The room was huge, cavernous. The teacher made the most of the space; she used it all, which meant she was usually calling to her students and their parents in a loud voice that got lost in the vast distance between her lips and our ears. I got used to repeating her instructions, but I wasn't always happy about it.

"If you're not going to pay attention, we're going to have to quit this class," became my mantra, but it made no difference. More often than not, Elizabeth went one way while everyone else went another, and I had to remind her of what the teacher had just said. In this case, I couldn't dismiss her behavior as a function of her age: in a class for children 18 months to 3 years, she was one of the oldest. There was another little girl in the class who was only a month older, and she did everything exactly when and as the teacher ordered.

I couldn't figure it out. At home and in music class, Elizabeth was obedient, well-behaved, chatty, and happy to participate in anything. At play school and gymnastics, she was either quiet and confused or dissolving into tears. Once again I found myself wondering what was wrong with my daughter, but this time I had an answer: maybe Dave had been right. Maybe she did have a hearing problem.

What made me finally take his concerns seriously was remembering a story that my mother had told me, years ago. It seems that at the end of my kindergarten year, the teacher called my mother and informed her that I was going to have to repeat the class.

"I was going to flunk kindergarten?" I said to my mother.

"You were going to be held back," she said.

Semantics, I thought to myself.

My mother wasn't about to let the teacher go ahead with her plan. "Why are you holding her back?" she wanted to know.

"She's immature," the teacher said. "She doesn't pay attention. She doesn't listen. She doesn't know how to follow directions."

My mother, who was also a kindergarten teacher, was aware that there were reasons other than immaturity that children might not pay attention in a classroom. "Have you had her hearing tested?" she asked.

"No," the teacher said.

"You don't hold her back until you have her hearing tested," my mother said.

My mother's instincts were right. I had a hearing loss, one that was corrected that summer when I underwent surgery to have my adenoids removed and tubes inserted in my eardrums to keep fluid from accumulating there and making it impossible for me to hear clearly. Instead of repeating kindergarten, I entered first grade that fall.

What surprised me more than the news that I was almost held back in kindergarten was that my own mother, who lived with me, hadn't detected my hearing loss sooner.

"We thought you weren't paying attention," she said.

At school, with near constant background noise, I wouldn't have heard much of anything, so my inattentiveness would have been consistent. At home, where it was quieter, I probably did hear much of what was going on, especially when whoever was addressing me was close by. When I didn't pay attention, my mother automatically assumed it was because I didn't want to listen.

How many times, I wondered, had I gotten scolded because I couldn't hear and my mother had misinterpreted it as defiance? How many times had I scolded Elizabeth and lost my temper with her because I thought she wasn't paying attention when, in fact, perhaps she couldn't hear?

I had no idea where to take Elizabeth for a hearing test, so I called one of my family doctors—the less busy one—for a recommendation. He insisted on examining Elizabeth first. As it turned out, so much wax was clogging her ear canals, he couldn't see through to her eardrums.

"Would impacted wax make it hard for her to hear?" I asked. He nodded.

I couldn't believe how relieved I felt. Once the wax came out, Elizabeth would be able to hear again! The temper tantrums would end! She'd be able to hear her gymnastics instructor!

"I'll make an appointment for you to see an audiologist," the doctor said, "but first we have to get this wax out."

I figured it would take a few minutes. Instead it took 3 weeks, during which Elizabeth had to have her ears flushed out four times and Dave and I had to put mineral oil in them every night to soften up the remaining wax.

During that time, she had her first hearing test. The clinic was close to our house, run by a husband-and-wife team. The wife had been an audiologist for a long time; the husband, a former schoolteacher, had only been practicing for a few years. For the purposes of this story, I'll call him Mike. He was a very nice man, and quite sweet to Elizabeth, but his inexperience showed, and it made me nervous.

Mike looked into Elizabeth's ears and then projected the enlarged image onto a screen so I could see. Her ear canal was now the diameter of an empty paper towel roll, and what it contained was neither pretty nor reassuring. Although her ears had been flushed out three times in the past 2½ weeks, gobs of wax remained, blocking any view of her eardrum.

"Will you be able to test her hearing?" I asked.

"We'll try," Mike said, although I could tell he wasn't confident.

He put a probe into Elizabeth's ear. The probe was connected to a wire that was connected to a little computer screen that displayed an empty graph. As we watched, a line stretched and squiggled across the graph. I had no idea what kind of test this was and what purpose it served, but I was so consumed with worry about Elizabeth's wax-filled ears that it didn't occur to me to ask. Also, it seemed as if Mike was having problems. He kept adjusting the probe and rerunning the test, but clearly he wasn't getting the results he expected. After trying nearly a half dozen times he summoned his wife into the room for help.

Months later, after umpteen trips to different audiologists, I learned that the test was called a tympanogram, and it's used to evaluate middle ear function. If the eardrum and middle ear are moving properly, the line will form a peak in the middle of the screen. If the middle ear contains fluid, which makes it difficult if not impossible for the eardrum to vibrate normally, the line will be flat.

Elizabeth's middle ears were filled with fluid, but I didn't know that at the time and, because the wax was blocking the view; neither did Mike. With his wife nearby, he tried the test once more. Then, with her blessing, he gave up and took Elizabeth into the sound booth for a hearing test. I stayed in the waiting area with Noah, who was awake and fidgety. After a short time, Mike brought Elizabeth back to the waiting room. The wax in her ears was making it impossible to get any usable results.

"Why don't you bring her back after her ears clear up?" he said. "We'll be able to do a thorough job then."

I figured that would be in another week. I was wrong. The next day, the doctor was able to flush the remaining wax out of Elizabeth's ears, but then he discovered she had "otitis media" in both ears.

I was shocked. Ear infections? My daughter? In the 33 months since she'd entered the world, Elizabeth had never, to my knowledge, had an ear infection. I'd always considered that an accomplishment of sorts. Besides, didn't kids who had ear infections scream, pull at their ears, and develop raging fevers to match the raging infections?

"Not all kids react the same way," the doctor said. "I'm going to give you some ear drops and a prescription for penicillin. Come back in 10 days, after the antibiotic's run its course, and we'll look at her ears again."

"Would an ear infection make it hard for her to hear?" I asked the doctor.

"The fluid in her ears certainly would," he said. "And it would make her uncomfortable, which could explain the tantrums."

Filled with hope that Elizabeth would soon be back to normal, I went off to the pharmacy to fill the prescriptions. Elizabeth took her medication dutifully. Her mood seemed slightly improved. Then, a little over a week later, on a Saturday morning, she woke up with pinprick red dots covering her torso.

"Is that chicken pox?" I asked Dave.

He had no idea, so we called our neighbor, Joan, a pediatrician. She wasn't our doctor—we'd never felt the need to have a pediatrician—but she was a friend, and she came over and inspected Elizabeth.

The verdict: either a virus or a reaction to the penicillin. We decided to go with the reaction-to-the-penicillin assessment and stopped giving it to her. The dots disappeared. The infection, on the other hand, lasted another 2 weeks.

The Monday after Joan examined Elizabeth, I tried to make an appointment with our regular doctor, to get a new prescription for Elizabeth. The doctor was sick and I didn't want to wait until he got better, so I was sent for the first time to a Dr. M., a pediatrician whose practice was nearby.

Dr. M.'s office was tiny and crammed full of children. The walls were covered with pictures of his patients, an inordinate number of whom, it seemed to me, were in wheelchairs or had unusual health problems. There were grateful letters from parents of children who had died, but had apparently benefited from Dr. M's loving care when they were living.

Dr. M. asked me to explain Elizabeth's situation. I told him the whole story, stopping occasionally to make sure he really needed all the details. He encouraged me to go on. When I finished, he asked me to get him a copy of the report from the audiologist.

"I don't think there is one," I said. Mike hadn't gotten any results worth recording; that's why he hadn't charged me and why he'd told me to come back when Elizabeth's ears were in better shape.

Two weeks later, Elizabeth's ear infection was gone, but Dr. M. told me not to schedule a hearing test. "Let's wait until her ears are cleared up," he said.

At the time, I didn't understand what he meant, nor did I feel the need or have the comfort level to ask for an explanation. Now I know fluid that accumulates in a child's ears because of a cold or an infection can linger for months. I also know that it's possible to have middle ear fluid without an infection.

At the end of December, about 10 weeks after the ear infection was diagnosed, Dr. M. examined Elizabeth and pronounced her healthy.

"Her ears are beautiful," he said.

Depending on my mood, I now consider his assessment bizarre, arrogant, ignorant, or amusing. At the time, I found it comforting.

"Should I take her back to the audiologist now?" I asked.

"Is she talking more?" he asked. "How's her behavior?"

"Great," I said. "She's doing really well."

"I wouldn't bother," he said.

"But she still isn't talking much," I pointed out. "And she's not always speaking clearly."

Speech therapy is available through our local public health clinic here in Edmonton, but according to Dr. M., there was a 6-month wait. "You could make an appointment," he said, "but most likely by the time she gets in, her speech will have cleared up."

To this day I'm not entirely sure why I didn't just take Elizabeth back to the audiology clinic right away. I didn't need Dr. M.'s referral: I already had an invitation to come back and finish what I'd started. But I didn't want to be a worry wart and I didn't want to take up the audiologist's precious time with my apparently baseless concerns when there were clearly other people with more serious needs.

True, Elizabeth had had a hearing problem—she'd had two, actually—but we'd cleared up both of them. There was no doubt she could hear better, and that her behavior had improved. Dave and I agreed there was no need to pursue this further; if the doctor said she was fine, she was fine.

But I couldn't get rid of the nagging, gnawing feeling that I had to see this thing through to its logical conclusion. I'd taken Elizabeth to the family doctor because I wanted her hearing tested by a professional. I still wanted that. But if the pediatrician, who clearly had far more experience with children than I, wasn't worrying, why should I?

At choir practice one night less than a week after Dr. M. had pronounced Elizabeth cured, I shared my concerns with a friend, a neonatal intensive care nurse who had worked with him in the past.

"Take Elizabeth to the audiologist, for your own piece of mind," she said.

I called Mike's office the next morning. It was the end of December. The next opening was February 1. Dave was going to be out of town, but that didn't worry me: I was going to bring Elizabeth to Mike, he was going test her and tell me her hearing was perfect, and I would go home knowing I'd followed through as planned.

Noah was asleep when we arrived at the clinic, and I was grateful, thinking I'd be able to watch the test undisturbed. Elizabeth and I followed Mike into the sound booth. I took a chair against the back wall and rested Noah on my lap. Elizabeth sat in front of me, her back to us. It was clear almost from the start that her hearing wasn't normal. When Noah woke up after a few minutes, it was even harder for me to ignore the truth: he consistently turned his head in whatever direction the sounds were coming from. Elizabeth stared straight ahead until the volume went up discernably.

*Say something!* I wanted to yell at her. *Respond! Tell the nice man you can hear the beeps! How could you not hear that beep? Why can't you hear that? I can hear it! Noah can hear it! Why can't you?*

I took Noah out of the room not long after. I told myself he was bored, squirming, and becoming a distraction, but deep down I know it's because I couldn't bear to see that my daughter couldn't hear sounds that were so obviously audible to the rest of the world.

Yet when Mike and his wife summoned me to a back office after Elizabeth's test, I was stunned when they told me the news: "Your daughter has a permanent hearing loss and will have to wear hearing aids for the rest of her life."

I felt as if I'd been told she had a terminal disease, not a correctable problem. Months later, when she had her first pair of hearing aids and her behavior and speech were noticeably improved, I wondered if my reaction might have been different if the news had been broken to me more gently, more positively. Perhaps if Mike and his wife had said, "Your daughter has a permanent hearing loss, and we know this because of how she reacted to all the tests we gave her, but she can be helped with hearing aids and we're going to find the best ones for her," I might not have felt so devastated. But all I could grasp was that my beautiful, lovely, healthy, perfect little girl was suddenly not so perfect. She was going to have hearing aids for the rest of her life, and who knew if that would help? What did I know about hearing aids, anyway? How could Mike and his wife be so sure they were right? They weren't doctors. Surely there was some operation that could fix her ears. They were wrong that the problem was permanent. I was certain they had made a mistake.

I couldn't bear to hear any more. I tried, unsuccessfully, to hold back the tears as Mike and his wife talked kindly to me about ear, nose, and throat specialists and having Elizabeth fitted for earmolds before the end of the week. I had no idea what an earmold was. I changed my mind a half dozen times in 2 minutes over whether to have Elizabeth fitted—whatever that meant—immediately, or to bring her back when Dave returned from his trip.

Mike and his wife were unfailingly patient. While I dithered about the earmold fitting, they tried to figure out which ear, nose, and throat doctor Elizabeth should see. Mike suggested one, and his wife said he'd retired. She suggested another one and he reminded her that the doctor was on vacation. I wasn't encouraged. By the time I left, they still hadn't given me a name, but that seemed the least of my worries.

I was literally halfway out the door with Elizabeth and Noah when I realized that almost nothing that Mike and his wife had said had sunk in. The sun had set and the office was closed; the receptionist had gone home for the day. I made my way back through the darkened waiting area to where Mike and his wife were doing their end-of-the-day chores. They didn't seem surprised to see me again so quickly, nor did my request strike them as unusual.

"I don't remember anything you just told me," I said. "I need a piece of paper, and I need you to tell me everything again, please, so I can write it down, so I won't forget."

# 2

# WHAT IS A HEARING LOSS?

On the way home from the clinic, I tried to conjure up an image of a child with hearing aids. I couldn't. I'd never seen one. Hearing aids were for old people, not children. Especially not little children. Especially not my perfect, beautiful little daughter.

I had a distant cousin who was deaf, the result of birth trauma. When I was growing up, my father had a colleague whose daughter lost her hearing after a childhood bout with meningitis. When she spoke, her voice was deep, flat, and nasal. The cousin didn't speak at all; she signed, beautifully. Her hands moved with a grace and lightness that made me think of butterflies.

But Elizabeth wasn't deaf. The audiologists had insisted on that, even when I tried to protest. "If she can't hear, she's deaf, isn't she?" I'd asked.

"She's hard of hearing," Mike and his wife had said gently. "A mild-to-moderate sensorineural hearing loss means she has some hearing."

It wasn't until months later, after Elizabeth began speech therapy at a local rehabilitation hospital, that I began to have a better understanding of how hearing loss works. Rachel, Elizabeth's speech pathologist, played a tape for Dave and me, to give us an idea of how and what a child with a mild-to-moderate loss such as Elizabeth's would hear. The words sounded muffled and chopped up. (See "Resources" for information on where you can hear similar recordings.) Rachel also gave us a picture from the Canadian Hearing Society, which provided an illustration of the difference between how sounds are perceived by people with normal hearing and how they are heard by those with hearing loss. People with normal hearing hear everything clearly. People with hearing loss hear fragments of sounds or, in some cases, no sound at all. Exactly what and how much they hear depends on the severity of the loss and how it affects the ability to perceive sound at various frequencies. What is consistent, despite the degree of loss, is that people with hearing loss don't hear as clearly as those with normal hearing. For example, without her hearing aids, Elizabeth might hear the word *some* as *thumb* or *table* as *able*.

What I didn't understand was how she could have developed *any* sort of a working vocabulary given that her loss apparently prevented her from hearing many of the individual sounds comprising speech, never mind sound blends such as *fl* and *sm*.

"You have a loud clear voice," Rachel reminded me. "That's a good thing—she was able to hear you. Your house is quiet, so that helped. And she has a mild-to-moderate loss, not one that's severe or profound."

At least if her loss were more serious, Dave and I would have been quicker to have had her tested, I thought, but there was no point continuing to torment myself about that. We'd figured out the problem; now we needed to understand and treat it.

Until I did some work as a broadcast journalist a few years before Elizabeth was born, I didn't give much thought to the technicalities of sound transmission. I knew the term dB, short for decibels, but only because it was the name of a rock band that was popular on the college circuit during the 1980s. I'd heard about sound waves and frequencies, but there was far too much physics involved for me to bother delving into either subject.

During my brief career at a radio station, I had no choice but to gain a greater insight into decibel levels and frequencies. That, combined with the audiogram, the graph used to show what a person can and can't hear, allowed me a basic understanding of Elizabeth's hearing loss. Especially helpful was an audiogram that showed the intensity and frequency level of various speech and environmental sounds (Figure 2-1).

There are two sets of numbers on the audiogram. The numbers on the left side of the chart denote decibel levels. The numbers across the top denote frequency levels.

Decibels are the units used to measure sound. Audiologists and others who work with these units use different decibel scales, depending how and for what purpose the units are used. The decibel scale depicted on an audiogram is *dB hearing level* (or dB HL),

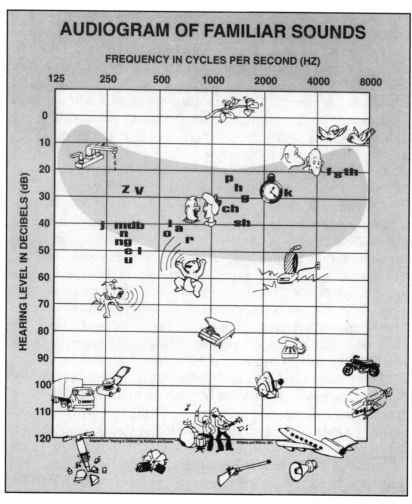

**Figure 2–1.** Audiogram of familiar sounds. Courtesy of the American Academy of Audiology.

which is used to represent the sound levels required to reach audibility. Nonprofessionals tend to use the familiar term, *loudness*, but loudness actually refers to the listener's subjective interpretation of intensity: that is, the greater the intensity of the sound, the louder it seems to the listener.

On an audiogram, the decibel hearing level ranges from 0 dB HL, a reference for the lowest (softest) sound level a young normal-hearing person can detect, to 120 dB HL, a very high-intensity sound.

Imagine sitting near the speakers at a rock concert and you'll have a sense of what 120 dB HL sounds like.

Frequency on an audiogram is measured in Hertz (for the 19th century German physicist Heinrich Hertz). It is abbreviated *Hz* and represents the rate of vibration (cycles per second) comprising the individual components of a given sound. We nonprofessionals like to use the more familiar term, *pitch*. Like loudness, pitch corresponds with the listener's subjective experience. High-pitch sounds are created when vibrations occur at a rapid rate. Low-pitch sounds occur when vibrations occur at a relatively slow rate. The higher the frequency, the higher in pitch it sounds to the listener.

For example, the key at the far left on a piano keyboard (it's an A, by the way) sends to your brain a signal that vibrates at approximately 28 cycles per second, or 28 Hz. It is the lowest note on the piano and for the normal hearing listener would be perceived as a very low-pitched sound. At the other end of the keyboard, on the far right, the key (a C) sends to your brain a signal that vibrates at approximately 4200 cycles per second, or 4200 Hz. It is the highest note on the keyboard and would be perceived by the listener as a very high-pitched sound. On most audiograms, frequencies range from a low of 250 Hz to a high of 8000 Hz.

Every person has hearing *thresholds*, the lowest decibel level their ears can detect. The threshold levels may differ across frequencies. For children, the normal range of hearing sensitivity is usually considered to be between 0 and 15 dB HL. For young adults, the normal range of hearing sensitivity is from 0 to 20 dB HL (Figure 2–2).

Children tend to have more sensitive hearing than adults because most have been spared the effects of exposure to high-intensity noise. Also, loss of hearing sensitivity, especially in the high frequencies, is a normal part of the aging process, so most older adults have some degree of hearing impairment.

---

### Audiogram Interpretation

*The audiogram is used to record the softest sounds (pure tones) a listener can detect, without amplification or a cochlear implant, at a range of test frequencies from low to high. The lowest level or* threshold *is recorded on the audiogram using the symbols in Figure 2–2. The normal range is at the top of the audiogram between 0 dB HL (the softest level a person with normal hearing can detect) up to about 20 dB HL. People with normal hearing have thresholds within this decibel range for all frequencies. Hearing losses in the 20 to 40 dB range are often described as mild, 41 to 55 dB as moderate, 56 to 70 dB as moderately severe, 71 to 90 as severe, and above 90 as profound (CDC, 2009). The region in the middle (see Figure 2–2) represents the sounds of speech. If your child's thresholds are* above *the speech region, she will be able to detect the sounds important for speech. If her thresholds are* below *the speech region, she will not hear any of the speech sounds. If her thresholds are* in or near *the speech region, she will hear some of the sounds important for speech. It may be helpful to plot your child's thresholds on an audiogram to get a better understanding of what sounds (if any) can be detected without amplification. Your audiologist can help with this.*

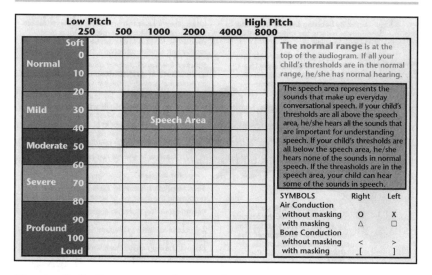

**Figure 2–2.** Pure tone audiogram. Courtesy of Robert Margolis, Ph.D., University of Minnesota.

However, the implications of a hearing loss present at birth are greater than they are in later years. Children need to hear the widest range of sounds necessary to develop proper speech and language skills. In contrast, an adult who has already acquired normal speech and language can better "fill in" the missing information. Of course, many adults require amplification too, but their problems are more specific to receptive communication; in other words, hearing aids help them to better hear what people are saying. For children still acquiring language, hearing aids are essential tools not only for hearing speech and language, but for developing and using speech.

When I was pregnant with Elizabeth, friends and magazine articles suggested I talk to my fetus. Apparently the more monologues I directed to my belly, the more comfortable the fetus would become with my voice. Once it was born, it would be that much more comfortable with me.

I couldn't bring myself to do it. Assuming it had normal hearing—and at that point I had no reason to assume otherwise—the fetus was going to hear me whether I talked directly to it or to my neighbor across the fence.

By the 19th or 20th week of gestation, a normally developing fetus can detect sound. But what's filtered through the womb is very different from what a baby will hear once she's out in the world. In the womb, sounds must pass through tissue and amniotic fluid. The normal tempo of speech is retained, but the higher pitches are reduced, making them sound lower in pitch.

If you want a sense of how a fetus hears, ask someone to talk to you with her face buried in a pillow. You'll hear sounds, but they will be low pitched and muffled. If you try really hard, you might be able to understand some of what you're hearing. However, given all that's blocking your sense of sound, you may feel you're better off conserving your energy. Interestingly, these *timing cues*, or rhythmic characteristics of speech, are important to a hard-of-hearing child once she enters the world, and can be vital to acquiring speech and language.

In terms of comprehension, you are far better off than the fetus. Although the unborn child can discern sounds, there is little hope of speech comprehension. The ability to make sense of language doesn't begin until after birth, when the brain has had weeks and months of exposure to sounds.

# How the Ear Works

The ear is divided into three parts: the outer ear, the middle ear, and the inner ear (Figure 2–3). The outer ear consists of the pinna, the visible part of the outer ear, and the ear canal, which leads to the eardrum. The ear canal contains hairs, as well as glands that produce wax, which is also known as cerumen. Both the hair and cerumen help keep debris away from the eardrum. The pinna and ear canal direct sound waves to the eardrum and the middle ear.

The eardrum is the dividing line between the outer ear and the middle ear. Inside the middle ear are three tiny bones: the malleus, the incus, and the stapes. One of the few facts I retained from junior high school biology is that those bones are also known as the hammer, the anvil, and the stirrup, which they closely resemble. The smallest bones in the body, the three comprise what is called the ossicular chain.

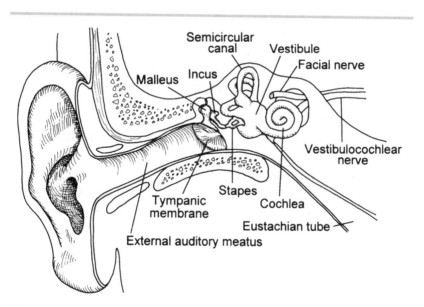

**Figure 2–3.** Anatomy of the ear. Note. From *Anatomy and Physiology for Speech, Language, and Hearing* (2nd ed., p. 566), by J. A. Seikel, D. W. King, and D. G. Drumright, 2000, San Diego, CA: Singular Publishing Group. Copyright 2000. Reprinted with permission.

The stapes, which is closest to the inner ear, is attached to the oval window, the membrane at the opening of the inner ear. Vibrations from the ossicular chain are transmitted to the fluids of the inner ear by movements of the stapes in and out of the oval window.

The fluid-filled inner ear consists of two parts: the semicircular canals, which are essential for balance, and the cochlea, which is the sensory organ for hearing. It is through the cochlea that nerve signals travel from the ear to the brain.

Cochlea is Latin for "snail." Contained within a bony chamber smaller than a pea, the cochlea is coiled two and a half times into the shape of a snail shell. Along the length of the fluid-filled cochlea is a membrane lined with microscopic hair cells that react to movements of the stapes in the oval window.

High frequencies stimulate the hair cells nearest the oval window. Low frequencies stimulate the hair cells at the far end of the cochlea, deep inside the coil. Most sounds we hear consist of many different frequencies at the same time. Because of that, the resulting pattern of vibration is highly complex.

In an ear that functions normally, sound waves traveling down the ear canal cause the eardrum to vibrate, which makes the bones of the ossicular chain vibrate, which stimulates the hair cells of the cochlea. The cochlea sends signals to the auditory nerve. The signals are transmitted to the brain, which interprets the sounds. These pathways develop early in life, after the brain has been exposed to sound.

One of the more disturbing pieces of information I kept coming across after Elizabeth's diagnosis was that the later a hard-of-hearing child is diagnosed and treated, the more likely he or she is to have speech and language delays. Presumably, the more severe the loss and the later the diagnosis and treatment, the more serious the delays. Studies have shown that some late-diagnosed children never catch up to their normal-hearing peers, although the effects of early identification and intervention are still under investigation.

Today, late is considered anything after about 6 months. That's a significant change from earlier years, when late was considered at or around 18 months. The most significant and tangible explanation for the change is technological. The development of hearing screening tests for newborns means that babies can be diagnosed soon after birth and fitted with hearing aids within the first weeks of life, or receive cochlear implants within 1–2 years of the diagnosis.

Being aided early and properly allows children to grow up developing age-appropriate speech and language skills. Most states in the United States and a growing number of provinces in Canada are committed to early screening and making it available for newborn infants.

By today's standards, Elizabeth was ancient by the time she was diagnosed at age 3. I did not appreciate the literature that warned me about the perils of late identification. As far as I could see, it was just more groundless fear-mongering designed to shake my already fragile faith in my parenting ability. But what was either missing or what I failed to glean is that there is an optimal period of time for children to learn speech and language, and the door is opened widest during the first 3 years of life. That's when most neural development occurs and language understanding begins.

I found it easiest to understand this phenomenon when it was explained in the context of someone learning a foreign language in high school: reading and understanding will come relatively easily, but you'll probably never speak like a native because you didn't learn the language at the most optimal time.

Similarly, children who have missed out on speech and language development because they couldn't hear properly may never learn to speak as well as those who have had that advantage. The less severe the hearing loss, the greater the chance the child will be able to successfully compensate. But the degree of loss is only one factor that will affect a child's speech and language development. Other factors that can and do make a difference are family support, speech and language stimulation, appropriateness of hearing aid fitting, maintenance of the hearing aids, and the child's learning style.

Seven months after Elizabeth was diagnosed she entered a preschool program for children with hearing loss. She had four classmates. The only other girl was a 3-year-old named Nikki, whom I'd heard about from Rachel, the speech-language pathologist. Nikki was born with a severe-to-profound high-frequency hearing loss in both ears.

Rachel was unabashedly impressed with Nikki's speech, vocabulary, and comprehension. "Her grandmother spends hours with her, reading, speaking, and practicing," she said. "It's unusual to find a 3-year-old with that degree of hearing loss who speaks as well as she does."

When I met Nikki and her grandmother, Gwen, and saw how they interacted, it became even clearer that Dave and I would play a significant role in helping Elizabeth make up for what she'd missed the past 3 years. With another toddler to care for, I didn't think I could spend the time Gwen did, making and laminating flashcards, reviewing worksheets, playing endless vocabulary games. What I could do was talk more. I began pointing out things I'd always considered obvious—"See how hard that doggie is panting! Look at all that sweat on his owner's face!"—and asking Elizabeth questions: "Why do you think they're so hot? I think they must have gone jogging. What do you think?"

"Children pick up a lot of language incidentally—not necessarily from conversation, but from what they hear around them," Rachel explained to me early on, when I discovered, much to my shock, that Elizabeth didn't understand concepts as basic as fast and high.

Like all children with hearing loss, she'd never had the advantage of being able to overhear. For her, simply hearing what was happening right in front of her was a challenge. As I discovered in the years immediately after she was aided, when presented with the opportunity to learn, she had no trouble. But where her younger brother seemed to increase his vocabulary simply by soaking up what he heard or overheard, with Elizabeth we had to be more active, pointing out words, providing definitions, and reinforcing what we'd just taught her.

## Hearing Loss: We've All
## Experienced It to Some Degree

Anyone who has ever had a head cold or impacted wax has no doubt experienced what's known as a conductive hearing loss, which is temporary and occurs when something prevents sound waves from being passed along to the inner ear. Causes can include otitis media (inflammation and fluid in the middle ear, which keeps the eardrum from vibrating properly) or an obstruction in the ear canal (from a buildup of cerumen, for example).

In either case, the inner ear is not affected. Sounds from the environment—music, other people's voices, traffic noises, rain falling on the roof—which must travel to the inner ear via the outer and middle ear pathway, are reduced in intensity, but as long as your cochlea is intact, you can still hear your own voice clearly. This is because some sounds can be conveyed directly to the inner ear fluids via *bone conduction*. The most common mode of bone conduction stimulation is a speaker's own voice. During speech, the movements of the larynx (voice box) send vibrations through the intervening bones and tissue, directly stimulating the fluids of the inner ear. As a result, people with conductive hearing loss have no problem hearing their own voice. However, outside sounds are reduced by the outer or middle ear disorder, resulting in a conductive hearing loss. Later in this book, I will discuss bone conduction testing performed by the audiologist as part of the hearing assessment.

In contrast to conductive hearing losses, which are usually temporary, sensorineural hearing losses are almost always permanent. Until Elizabeth was diagnosed, I'd never heard the word *sensorineural*. At the time I was so overwhelmed by the idea that she had a permanent hearing loss that I didn't stop to think about how sensible a term it is. "Sensory" refers to inner ear function, and "neural" refers to the auditory nerve. Most permanent losses are due to sensory (inner ear) dysfunction: a malformation in the cochlea; or hair cells that never developed, don't work properly or developed but were then destroyed. A small percentage of children with sensorineural hearing loss have a problem with transmission of sound from the inner ear to the auditory nerve, the nerve itself, the higher auditory pathways, or some combination of these conditions. Although the condition itself is not new, advances in diagnostic audiology procedures have made it possible to identify these children as having *auditory neuropathy*. Auditory neuropathy results in dysfunction of the auditory nerve or higher auditory pathway, while inner ear (sensory) function remains intact. The incidence has not been clearly established, but estimates range from 7 to 10% of all infants with congenital sensorineural hearing loss (see Info Box).

The more common sensory hearing losses may be due to one or more of the conditions described later in this chapter (see Info Box), but it's important to remember that these conditions do not always result in hearing loss. Elizabeth didn't seem to fit into any of the known categories, and for the first 2 years after she was diagnosed, I spent a lot of time—too much, probably—trying to come up with an explanation.

The audiology clinic where we eventually went for her hearing aids had a lot of pediatric patients. On any given visit we were likely to see at least one other child. One morning I got into a discussion with the parents of a girl who was a little younger than Elizabeth and had been wearing hearing aids since around her first birthday.

---

**Auditory Neuropathy**

*Children with auditory neuropathy have a hearing disorder that causes difficulty understanding speech and other sounds because of a disturbance in the transmission of signals from the inner ear to the brain. The condition has also been called* auditory dyssynchrony. *It usually affects both ears.*

*Some children with auditory neuropathy benefit from amplification; others do not. Those who are not helped by amplification often obtain benefit from a cochlear implant, perhaps because electrical stimulation helps to synchronize the auditory system. It is important to note that this condition is highly variable; that is, the severity of auditory neuropathy ranges from mild to severe. In 2008, an international guidelines development panel recommended the terminology* auditory neuropathy spectrum disorder *to emphasize the variability of the condition and its affects on communication.*

*Young children with auditory neuropathy are best served by a team of specialists including an otologist, audiologist, and early intervention providers. See "Resources" for further information.*

---

Her parents had to watch her constantly to make sure she didn't drop them into their coffee or the toilet bowl. She had a much more severe loss than Elizabeth; her speech was incomprehensible to me.

"Did you go for genetic testing?" I asked them.

They looked at me as if I were nuts. "No," they said, the unspoken message being, "Our child can't hear. Her situation can't get much worse. We have more important things to think about."

## Searching for the Cause

For the first time, I wondered if my search for an explanation was a trivial luxury that was keeping me from dealing with the real problem. Maybe it was—but it didn't stop me. Other people had explanations. Didn't we deserve one?

Nikki, Elizabeth's preschool classmate, inhaled a mixture of meconium and amniotic fluid at birth, which severely compromised her oxygen levels. The hair cells of the inner ear crave oxygen. When Nikki was born, her hair cells, deprived of oxygen, stopped working. To date, no one has come up with a way to regenerate hair cells in humans, although scientists have discovered evidence of hair cell regeneration in chickens. At least for the time being, however, the loss of cochlear hair cells in humans means a permanent loss of hearing.

Could Elizabeth's hearing loss have been caused by birth trauma? I posed the question to Dr. Elliott, the ear, nose, and throat specialist we saw a week after her initial diagnosis. I was induced 2½ weeks before my due date because of high blood pressure. Elizabeth's heart rate plunged even before I went into labor, necessitating an emergency C-section. But she was fine when she eventually emerged; she did so well that my doctor granted both of us permission to leave the hospital a day early.

No, Dr. Elliott said, he doubted her hearing loss had anything to do with the circumstances of her birth.

Becky, who lives across the street from us and is a year younger than Elizabeth, also has a high-frequency loss, though not as severe as Nikki's. Becky's parents initially thought her loss may have been caused by Gentamycin, an antibiotic she received intravenously, first when she was born with a collapsed lung that the doctors initially diagnosed as pneumonia, and then 3 months later when she developed a high fever from a bladder infection.

Kathy, Becky's mom, didn't know that Gentamycin can be ototoxic (harmful to the ear). Even if she had, she might not have protested. "If you're staring at a child who, you're being told, could have pneumonia, would you withhold that drug?" she asked.

Tests eventually showed the Gentamycin hadn't caused Becky's hearing loss. Her parents still don't have an explanation. I, meanwhile, pressed on. Was it the antibiotic ear drops Elizabeth had been prescribed to fight the ear infection we discovered when she was 2½, I asked Dr. Elliott? No, he said. Those drops wouldn't have gotten past her eardrum; they'd been nowhere near her inner ear or her bloodstream.

Dr. Elliott sent Dave, Elizabeth, and me to our local university's genetics clinic for testing, which also turned up nothing. He sent Elizabeth for a CT scan, which he said had a 20% chance of showing an abnormality of the inner ear. All it showed was that she had fluid in her middle ears. No surprise there: at the time of the CT scan, she was recovering from a cold. We'd known she had fluid in her ears. On the other hand, the test also showed that her bone structure was normal. In one sense, it was a relief; at least there was nothing wrong with her bone structure. But it was yet another source of frustration: how were we ever going to figure out what *had* caused the problem?

"For most children who have permanent hearing loss, there is no explanation," Dr. Elliot stated during our first visit, but every time I came up with another possibility, I brought it to him.

Dr. Elliot had a 6-month waiting list and no partner with whom to share the patient load, and his small office was once so crowded that Elizabeth and I opted to wait in a nearby donut shop. Yet he seemed to have endless patience for what another physician might have considered mindless, irritating questions.

It was after I wondered, for perhaps the 10th or 11th time, if Elizabeth might have lost her hearing because of a high fever, that I quit asking. Maybe it was Dr. Elliot's answer—that an audiogram such as Elizabeth's was usually a sign of a malformation deep in the cochlea, one that can't be detected. Or maybe I'd just come to the same conclusion as that family of the little girl in the audiology clinic: My daughter can't hear very well, but lucky for us, it looks as if her hearing isn't getting any worse.

Scientists have begun to identify a number of recessive genes that may be associated with hearing loss. Recessive genetic inheritance occurs when two normal hearing parents have the same abnormal gene for hearing. The parents are unaffected because they also have a *dominant* gene for normal hearing. But when two people match up the same abnormal hearing gene, they have a one-in-four chance of having a child with hearing loss. Screening is now performed only for the more common genetic abnormalities, among them a mutation called connexin 26, which is responsible for one third of all cases of genetic hearing loss.

The summer after Elizabeth turned 6, when I had completed a draft of this chapter for our first edition that concluded with, "Even as I write this, I am confident that in a lab somewhere, someone is trying to figure out what causes losses like Elizabeth's," we got a call from the genetics clinic we'd visited when she was first diagnosed.

"We've started testing for connexin 26," the genetics counselor, Karin, said to me. "Would you like to have Elizabeth tested?"

## Causes of Hearing Loss in Children

*The causes of permanent hearing loss in young children include both genetic (inherited) and acquired conditions. Genetic causes are now believed to account for about half of all hearing loss present at birth. Nongenetic causes account for about one fourth. The cause of the remaining one fourth is unknown. Within the half known to be genetically linked, nearly three fourths are due to a form of inheritance called* autosomal recessive, *which occurs when each parent has an abnormal gene for hearing. This results in a one-in-four chance of the child being born with hearing loss. Other types of genetic inheritance can occur when only one parent has an abnormal gene.*

*There are many causes of* nongenetic *(acquired) hearing loss in young children. Sensorineural hearing loss has been associated with medications that damage the ear and with infections and illnesses that occur at birth or later, including meningitis, measles, mumps, and some neurological diseases.*

*Hearing loss can also occur as part of a syndrome or* sequence. *These are collections of signs or symptoms that occur together indicating a particular disease or condition that may be genetic or nongenetic in origin. Some of the more common syndromes and sequences that include permanent hearing loss are Usher syndrome, Treacher-Collins syndrome, Pendred syndrome, CHARGE association, and Waardenberg syndrome. For most syndromes the hearing loss is present at birth, but some, such as Turner syndrome, have a later onset. See "Resources" for additional information on these and other conditions.*

Dave, who will do anything to avoid contact with a needle, didn't think we should bother. The chances that Elizabeth would test positive were slim, and besides, hadn't we already accepted that we would never know the cause of her hearing loss, that what was important wasn't finding a cause but dealing with the problem?

"She likes hospitals," I reminded him. "Besides, they've offered, and it's free. We might as well do it. Maybe we'll learn something."

Elizabeth had an appointment at the genetics clinic in early fall. She missed half a morning at school, answering the geneticists' questions, standing and sitting patiently, and finally heading down to the blood lab where she impressed the technician with her ability to remain still while her blood was drawn into little vials. Nearly 2 months later, in mid-November, Karin called to tell me Elizabeth had tested positive for two mutations on the connexin 26 gene.

To this day I can't believe my reaction: I was elated. I felt as if I'd won a lottery. I could barely keep my feet on the ground or my voice from shouting for joy. Apparently learning the root cause had been more important to me than I'd wanted to admit. Yet, with the exception of the rare instances when someone asks how Elizabeth lost her hearing, the test results have had no discernable effect on our daily lives.

Research has shown that most connexin 26 hearing losses tend to be stable, but we'd already suspected Elizabeth's hearing loss isn't progressive. None of our relatives have been tested, although they've been offered the opportunity. As for Noah, we don't know if he is a carrier: the genetics clinic won't test him until he's old enough to decide for himself.

After the initial excitement of the news wore off, I felt guilty all over again—Elizabeth *had* been hard of hearing at birth, and we *had* missed it. But those feelings diminished quickly: the time for tormenting myself was long past. Better to use my energy for more important things, like helping Elizabeth get the most out of the hearing she has, and out of life in general.

# 3

# ASSESSMENT AND INTERVENTION

When Elizabeth was a baby, in 1996, I would take her to our local health clinic for immunizations. That's standard practice here in Edmonton, the Canadian city where I live. It was also standard practice for the public health nurse to ring a bell at some time during these visits, presumably to see if Elizabeth could hear. She always turned to look at the bell. In other words, she passed the test, something I'd completely forgotten until I brought Noah in for his last immunization when he was 5 and Elizabeth almost 7. I didn't see a bell anywhere.

"Do you still ring a bell to test hearing?" I asked the nurse.

She shook her head. "We were told to stop," she said. "It didn't work. Now we ask the parent questions, and if there's any sign of a hearing loss, we recommend following up with an audiologist."

To be fair, our public health nurses aren't the only ones who once thought the best way to test hearing was to make a loud noise and observe the child's reaction. I've heard from countless parents whose pediatricians and even ear, nose, and throat specialists have employed this crude method.

The reason it's so popular is that it's simple and the results appear indisputable. But no matter how effective it may look, it's never going to be accurate because people are sensitive to motion. If we sense movement, we'll turn in that direction regardless of what we hear. People with hearing loss are especially attuned to visual cues in the environment. Another reason crude noise tests can be misleading is that a child with a high-frequency hearing loss, with normal or near-normal low-frequency hearing, may respond consistently to speech and other sounds while much of the high-frequency information is missing.

Whenever there is any question about hearing an audiologist should conduct a thorough assessment, especially in a young child. I'll say more about audiology and audiologists later in this chapter.

## Identification of Hearing Loss and Middle Ear Problems

Hearing screening tests are designed to identify children who are at risk for hearing loss; that is, children who should be referred for diagnostic assessment by an audiologist. Diagnostic tests are used to determine the type and extent of the hearing problem—whether it's permanent or a disorder that can be corrected, such as impacted wax (cerumen) or fluid (effusion) behind the eardrum. With young children there can be a combination of permanent and temporary causes. The nature of the problem will determine what referrals and intervention are needed.

Newborn hearing screening requires *physiologic tests*; that is, tests that can be administered without the baby's active participation. In contrast, *behavioral tests* require the child to respond in some repeatable way to sounds presented from a loudspeaker or earphone. Because behavioral tests are not reliable until babies reach a developmental age of about 6 months, newborn hearing screening is conducted using physiologic tests. Although physiologic tests do not provide a direct measure of hearing, they can be used to identify hearing loss in an infant or young child.

## Newborn Hearing Screening

In several Canadian provinces and nearly all states in the United States, newborns are screened for hearing loss at birth, before being discharged from the hospital. At the time of this writing, in Canada the provinces requiring universal screening were Prince Edward Island, New Brunswick, Ontario, and British Columbia. In other provinces newborn screening is offered for at-risk infants and at some hospitals when parents request it, but it is not mandatory. For information about screening programs in the United States, see http://www.ncham.org, which provides a summary of policies and procedures for each state.

Two technologies are used for newborn screening: otoacoustic emissions (OAEs) and the auditory brainstem response (ABR). For either test the ideal scenario is a sleeping baby. Newborns can be screened in natural sleep but older infants or toddlers often require sedation.

## Otoacoustic Emissions

OAEs are low-intensity sounds produced by the inner ear, specifically, the outer hair cells of the cochlea. They are detected by a sensitive microphone placed in the ear canal (Figure 3–1). Successful recording of OAEs means there is both a healthy inner ear (cochlea) and normal or near-normal middle ear function. OAEs are said to be *preneural* because they occur only at the level of the cochlea. This makes it possible to evaluate the cochlea without involving higher levels of the auditory system. The sounds used to produce an OAE may be clicks or tones. When OAEs can be measured, it usually means normal hearing sensitivity or no more than a mild hearing loss. But absent OAEs can result from a variety of conditions ranging from middle ear fluid to profound cochlear hearing loss. Other tests are needed to determine why OAEs are absent. OAE screening may be conducted by a variety of professionals including nurses and pediatricians. Diagnostic OAE testing is usually conducted by an audiologist as part of a diagnostic test battery.

## The Auditory Brainstem Response

As with OAEs, the ABR is produced by presenting clicks or tones through a probe in the ear canal. What's different is that responses are recorded from small electrodes attached to the head (Figure 3–2). The responses provide information about the function of the auditory nerve and the auditory pathway through the brainstem. No electricity is delivered to the child. Rather, the ABR equipment detects and amplifies the tiny electrical (neural) events that occur in

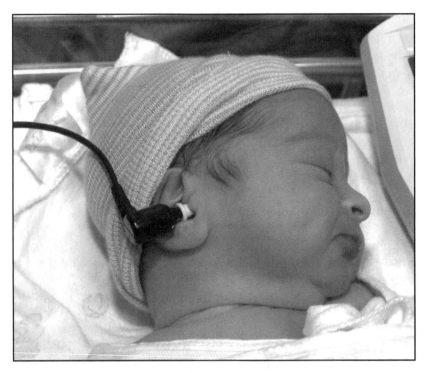

**Figure 3–1.** Newborn hearing screening with otoacoustic emissions. Courtesy of Jackson Roush, University of North Carolina School of Medicine.

response to the test sounds. Unlike OAEs, which are usually present or absent, the ABR test can be used to estimate the amount of hearing loss across a range of frequencies. As noted earlier, ABR can be used for screening in the newborn nursery. Audiologists use more advanced ABR tests to obtain the information needed to diagnose hearing loss and begin the process of hearing aid selection and fitting.

Both OAE and ABR are used for newborn hearing screening. For babies with uncomplicated pregnancy and delivery, either technology is fine. But for infants who required more than a few days in the neonatal intensive care unit (NICU) the Joint Committee on Infant Hearing recommends that hearing screening be performed only with ABR because of the increased risk of auditory neuropathy (see Info Box).

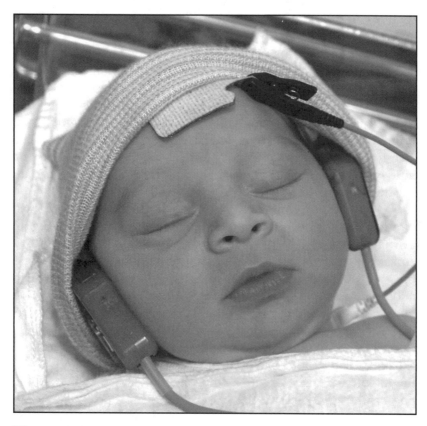

**Figure 3–2.** Newborn hearing screening with auditory brainstem responses. Courtesy of Jackson Roush, University of North Carolina School of Medicine.

## Hearing and Middle Ear Screening for Older Children

For older children, routine hearing screening is often done by a nurse or other health care professional. It usually begins with a visual inspection of the outer ear for noticeable signs of disease, malformation, or other abnormality. This is followed by an *otoscopic inspection*, which involves examining the ear canal and eardrum (the eardrum is also known as the *tympanic membrane*). This requires an otoscope, an instrument that functions as both a light and a magnifier.

It's not unusual for a child to balk at the idea of having the oto-scope tip inserted into the ear canal. If that happens, the person performing the exam may be willing to take some time to explain what the instrument is and how it's used. You can hold your child on your lap if it makes him feel safer and helps to keep him still. If he's brought along a stuffed animal or doll, you can ask the clini-cian to provide a demonstration using the animal or doll. Taking a little extra time to make your child comfortable can save time and frustration over the long haul.

Once the otoscopic inspection is complete, the clinician will often screen for otitis media (fluid behind the eardrum) using an instrument called a tympanometer. A soft probe tip, similar in size and appearance to the OAE probe, is inserted into the ear canal and pressure changes are made to determine how the eardrum and middle ear respond. The test doesn't hurt and only takes a few sec-onds, but your child must be still so your lap may be needed again.

The tympanometer prints out a graph illustrating how the eardrum and middle ear are working. There is supposed to be a small air-filled chamber behind the eardrum. When there is air in the middle ear space—that is, when the middle ear is functioning properly—the tracing on the graph will form a "peak," like a hill that narrows at the top. If the eustachian tube isn't functioning well because of allergies, cold, or an upper respiratory infection, the test may indicate negative pressure in the middle ear space. The most likely outcome when there is *fluid* behind the eardrum is a "flat" tracing. Although this is usually a temporary condition, the fluid adds additional *conductive* hearing loss to the underlying per-manent hearing loss. Needless to say, the last thing a hard-of-hearing child needs is additional loss due to otitis media. That's why it's important to have regular middle ear monitoring. For example, your pediatrician will probably use the otoscope to check your child's ears at each visit. Your audiologist is likely to obtain a tympanogram with each assessment. You should seek a medical opinion and hear-ing assessment any time you feel there may be a change in your child's hearing or if you suspect other symptoms of otitis media. It's important to keep in mind that otitis media can occur even in the absence of ear pain or other symptoms.

## Otitis Media

*Otitis media, an inflammation of the middle ear, is one of the most common diseases of early childhood. An ear infection, which usually results in an earache and fever, occurs when there is infected fluid in the middle ear. Pediatricians call this* acute otitis media *and they often choose to treat it with antibiotics. It is possible to have middle ear fluid without infection. This is called* otitis media with effusion *(OME). When a child has OME there are no symptoms other than hearing loss due to the blockage created by the middle ear fluid. This hearing loss is temporary and goes away once the fluid has absorbed or drained, which can take up to 6 weeks. To insure good health and optimal hearing, children with sensorineural hearing loss should be routinely screened for otitis media.*

*When there is a history of chronic or frequent OME, the physician may recommend* pressure equalization tubes, *referred to by most lay people as* PE tubes. *Tube placement is a routine medical procedure performed by an ENT specialist with the child under general anesthetic. PE tubes provide a consistent airway from the ear canal to the middle ear space, maintaining equal air pressure on both sides of the eardrum. The tubes rarely need to be removed; they are designed to work their way out after a few months. Children with chronic middle ear problems may require several sets of tubes.*

## Behavioral Hearing Assessment

As noted earlier, behavioral testing requires the listener's participation. Almost all of us have had some experience with behavioral hearing screening. When I was in elementary school in the 1960s, the school district's audiologist set up shop in our gym a couple of times a year. Armed with a portable audiometer—a machine designed to emit sounds at varying frequency and decibel levels—he'd fit a cumbersome pair of headphones over my ears and deliver a series of beeps. My job was to tell him which ear heard the sounds.

Based on my antiquated experience, I thought I knew what Elizabeth would go through when she had her hearing tested. But technology had come a long way in the more than 30 years between our tests. The sleek sound booths in the Edmonton audiology clinics I have visited with Elizabeth are considerably more sophisticated than what the Utica Public Schools had at their disposal back in the 1960s and early 1970s.

Elizabeth's first hearing tests fell into the category of *pure-tone audiometry*. She had to identify which ear was hearing a high-, medium-, or low-pitched beep presented through earphones at varying decibel levels. Elizabeth was always cooperative at her hearing tests: she was an ideal, agreeable patient. Not all children are. In fact, I've heard about behavioral assessments taking weeks or even months to complete. It took my neighbor's daughter, Becky, 6 months to get a diagnosis.

"Becky was really scared," her mom, Kathy, says. That's because before she even made it to the audiologist, she'd had a handful of other traumatic medical experiences. She'd had significant amounts of wax flushed out of her ears with a large metal syringe. She'd had visits with other specialists at the same hospital where the audiologist was located. In the course of testing her for a syndrome similar to muscular dystrophy, one doctor "came at her with a huge foot-long reflex hammer, and that just sent her around the bend," Kathy recalls. "These things were not helping. They were taking place at the same site as the hearing test. Every time we pulled up to the parking lot, she'd refuse to get out of the car."

Kathy began scheduling the audiology appointments further and further apart. "Each time, Becky would be completely noncompliant and lay on the floor in a ball," she says. "I thought we were wasting our time, and I was damaging our child emotionally. I didn't want it to be a traumatic experience, so we kept on lengthening the time between the visits."

At each visit, Kathy and the audiologist tried something new— toys, stickers, games. What finally made a difference was bringing in another child, Becky's 6-year-old cousin, to model the correct testing behavior. When Becky saw her cousin sitting through the hearing test, apparently experiencing no pain, she was willing to try, too. "She saw it was safe, it was okay, and she could do it," Kathy says. "We finally got some testing completed, and she was more and more compliant as we went along."

Nowadays it's not necessary to delay the intervention process when children are difficult to test. Although older infants and toddlers require sedation for ABR and other diagnostic tests, in the long run it is much more efficient and easier on both the child and parents to complete the testing as soon as possible.

While OAE and ABR provide important information regarding the auditory system, behavioral tests provide the most detailed information regarding hearing thresholds and the type and degree of hearing loss. The first behavioral test, visual reinforcement audiometry (VRA), can be administered when the child reaches a developmental age of about 6 months. For this test the infant is seated in a high chair or, more commonly, on a parent's lap while the audiologist presents tones at different frequencies and intensities. When the baby turns toward the loudspeaker emitting the sound, he is rewarded with a flashing light and moving toy (the visual reinforcement) near the loudspeaker. Eventually, most children will allow small insert earphones to be placed in their ears (Figure 3–3), making it possible to observe responses from each ear. Since testing with tones from a loudspeaker does not allow sounds to be delivered to each ear separately, it provides a measure of "better ear" sensitivity.

Eventually most children are able to be tested using *play audiometry*, a method of testing that allows a child to respond by dropping a block or performing some other play activity when the sound is heard. Sometimes the audiologist will use a combination of VRA and play audiometry. The goal is to determine a threshold at each frequency, that is, the softest level a child can detect at each frequency.

VRA and play audiometry, as described here, involve presenting *air conduction* sounds, those that travel through the air before they arrive at the eardrum. The audiologist is also interested in how the inner ear responds (that is, a response without the participation of the middle ear). This is accomplished by stimulating the inner ear directly with a bone vibrator (Figure 3–4).

A comparison of responses to air- and bone-conducted sounds allows the audiologist to determine not only how much hearing loss there is at each frequency, but whether part of the loss is due to a middle ear problem such as otitis media. Eventually a complete

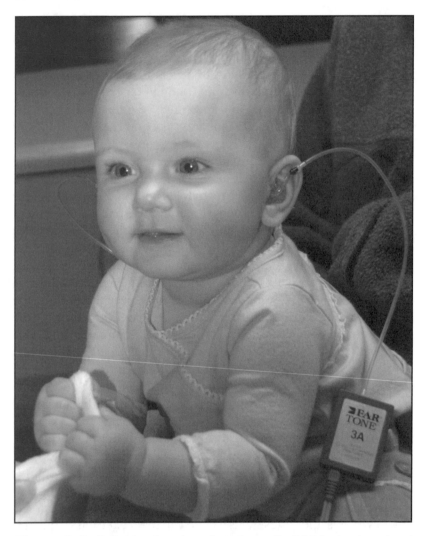

**Figure 3–3.** Behavioral testing of an 8-month-old infant using visual reinforcement audiometry. Note insert receivers attached to the child's custom earmolds. Courtesy of Jackson Roush, University of North Carolina School of Medicine.

picture will emerge, making it possible to construct an audiogram, the graph that shows hearing sensitivity for each frequency (see Chapter 2).

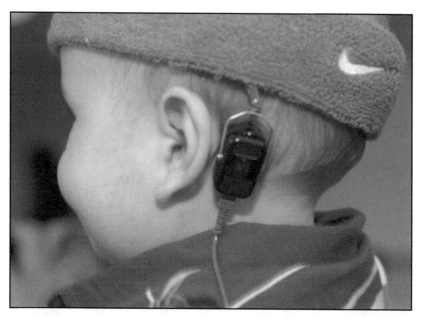

**Figure 3–4.** A bone vibrator is used to deliver sound signals directly to the inner ear, bypassing the middle ear. Hearing by *bone conduction* is then compared to responses obtained from an earphone to determine the type of hearing loss. Courtesy of Jackson Roush, University of North Carolina School of Medicine.

Your child will undergo many behavioral tests. In the early years the purpose of this will be to accurately define the type and degree of hearing loss. Later it will be important to provide monitoring to determine whether the loss is stable or changing.

## How Much Information Is Needed

The goal of the hearing test is to obtain a detailed assessment of hearing sensitivity for each ear. It is important to emphasize that a complete diagnostic picture is not needed in order to proceed with hearing aid selection and fitting. I have heard from parents whose referral to the audiologist was delayed for weeks or even months.

A diagnostic ABR test performed by a pediatric audiologist will provide sufficient information (accurate predictions of low- and high-frequency hearing sensitivity) to proceed with hearing aid selection and fitting. Over time additional information will be added making it possible to refine the hearing aid fitting. It should be noted that hearing aid fitting is usually the first step even for children who will later receive cochlear implants.

## Specialists in Your Life

In most families, the child's primary health care provider is a pediatrician. Once a child is diagnosed with permanent hearing loss, the pediatrician becomes one member of a team of health care and educational professionals. If your family decides to use a spoken language approach, you and your child may work with a speech-language pathologist (SLP), an auditory-verbal (AV) therapist, a teacher of deaf and hard-of-hearing children, or a combination of specialists. Depending on the degree of hearing loss and the communication method you choose, your child may also need an interpreter, a translator, or a transliterator. If your child has other disabilities or health problems (and many do), there will be even more professionals involved.

Your priorities and your child's needs will determine the members of the team. There may be personnel changes along the way. If your health insurance provider or school district is resistant to covering necessary services, or if you feel their services are insufficient, you will need to advocate for your child. (See Chapter 9.)

### Pediatric Audiologist

An audiologist is a hearing health care professional with a master's degree or a professional doctorate (AuD) from an accredited university program. All students now entering audiology programs in the United States earn an AuD. Students entering audiology programs in Canada are expected to earn a master's degree, which is the minimum needed to practice.

> ### When Hearing Loss Occurs with Other Disabilities
>
> *Studies have shown that nearly 40% of children with permanent hearing loss have one or more disabilities in addition to hearing loss. These conditions range from mild learning problems to severe disabilities. According to a survey by the Gallaudet Research Institute, the most common conditions that occur with hearing loss include learning disabilities, intellectual disabilities, attention disorders, visual impairment, and cerebral palsy.*
>
> *If you feel your child has an undiagnosed disability in addition to hearing loss, it is important to share your concerns with your pediatrician and other service providers. Referral to a specialist or evaluation by a multidisciplinary team may be needed to determine if the condition is present and, if so, the best treatment or course of action.*

Audiologists are educated in the functions of the ear, how to determine if there's a hearing loss, and what to do when there is. Although other professionals may conduct hearing screening and other tests, when there is any doubt about a child's hearing, the test should be conducted by a pediatric audiologist.

It is important to understand that not all audiologists have experience with infants and young children. I strongly recommend that you try to find one who does, and who enjoys working with them. The Web sites of the American Academy of Audiology (http://www .audiology.org), the American Speech-Language-Hearing Association (http://www.asha.org), and the Canadian Association of Speech-Language Pathologists and Audiologists (CASLPA; http://www.cas lpa.ca) include directories of member audiologists (see Resources). CASLPA lists only private practitioners who wish to be listed. If members have specified that they work with pediatric patients, that information is included. Your pediatrician, primary care physician, or other professionals may also be able to help you find an audiologist who works with young children. As you meet other

parents, they too will be helpful. Finding a well-qualified and experienced pediatric audiologist, even if it means traveling some distance, is well worth the effort.

## Pediatrician or Primary Care Physician

The pediatrician or primary care physician will continue to address
your child's general medical needs. After the diagnosis of hearing
loss, his responsibilities will include referral to appropriate specialists. Keep in mind that even pediatricians who have been practicing
for years may have limited experience with permanent hearing loss.
Make sure the other professionals keep your pediatrician informed
and up to date regarding your child's hearing loss and its management, and make sure you are on everyone's mailing lists as well.

## Otolaryngologist

Any child suspected of having a permanent hearing loss should be
examined by an otolaryngologist. A specialist in diagnosing and treating the ear, nose, throat, and related disorders of the head and neck,
an otolaryngologist is also known as an *ENT*. Those who specialize
in ears are called *otologists*.

The ENT examination is essential to ensure that your child
receives a comprehensive diagnosis. In addition to checking for middle ear problems, the ENT will check for other medical problems.
This is important because, as noted earlier, some children with congenital hearing loss have one or more other conditions that may be
associated with illness or other disabilities.

If your child suffers from chronic otitis media with effusion
(OME), which further degrades his hearing, the ENT may perform
minor surgery to insert pressure equalization tubes (PE-tubes) in
the eardrum. If your child needs a cochlear implant, an otologist
will provide the surgery. As with any professional who will work
with your child, it's best if you can find an ENT who specializes in
pediatrics. The ENT will also help determine the need for referral
to other medical specialists in ophthalmology (eyes) or neurology,
or to a genetic counselor for families who want that information.

## Geneticist/Genetic Counselor

A geneticist is a health care professional (MD or PhD) with special training in genetics, the study of heredity. Over half of all permanent hearing loss in children is hereditary. Sometimes it is part of a syndrome, which means that other medical abnormalities are present. If your pediatrician, primary care physician, or ENT cannot determine a cause for your child's hearing loss, you will probably want to consult with a geneticist. If a genetic cause is found, it can spare you and your child from other diagnostic procedures. You can also find a geneticist on the National Society of Genetic Counselors Web site (http://www.nsgc.org/).

The geneticist may work with a genetic counselor (a certified professional who usually has a master's degree or PhD) who can explain the genetic reasons for hearing loss, take a family history, and help you decide whether you or your child should be tested. If a test is done, the counselor can explain the results and put you in touch with other resources.

The geneticist will review your child's medical records and your family history, examine your child for signs of a syndrome, suggest appropriate medical tests, and explain the results of genetic testing.

Genetic testing usually requires a blood test, although some doctors will test a piece of skin. The sample is sent to a lab, which runs tests to determine if there are changes or mutations that can cause a hearing loss. It may take several weeks to complete the test.

If testing reveals the cause of your child's hearing loss, the geneticist or genetic counselor may also be able to tell you whether your child is likely to have or develop additional health problems, and whether the hearing loss is likely to be progressive or remain stable. You and your spouse may also be tested. If you are planning to have more children, the geneticist may be able to tell you the likelihood of those children being born with a hearing loss. If your child's hearing loss is part of a syndrome, the geneticist may be able to refer you to a support group or provide additional information.

Genetics is an evolving science. The most common cause for childhood hearing loss not related to a syndrome is a mutation in a gene called *connexin 26*. Tests for that mutation didn't exist until the 1990s. If your child has genetic testing and the test results are inconclusive, don't despair. Eventually there may be a test that will provide an answer. In the meantime remember that genetic tests provide information, not a cure. A geneticist cannot fix your child's hearing. But having a better understanding of the underlying cause can be helpful, and also useful for planning purposes. Some day your child may also be interested in this information.

## Ophthalmologist

An ophthalmologist is a physician and surgeon who specializes in treating diseases and disorders of the eye and optic nerve. A child with a hearing loss obviously needs optimal vision. The Joint Committee on Infant Hearing in the United States recommends that children with hearing loss have an ophthalmology exam. Regular monitoring should be provided to rule out late-onset vision disorders that might be associated with hearing loss. The ophthalmologist will tell you how often a reexamination should be provided based on your child's history. Of course, an eye examination should be scheduled any time you have concerns about your child's vision.

## Communication Options

For the parents of a child newly identified with hearing loss, choosing a communication method can be frustrating and bewildering. Professionals are understandably devoted to their preferred methods of communication, and getting unbiased information is not always easy. In reality the choices may be limited, especially in a small town or rural area. Still, it's important to know about the various communication options and to choose the method best suited for your family. It's also important to remember that you can change your mind. What may seem optimal at one point in time may change as you learn more and as your child develops. Following is a brief description of each communication method. Additional information on each can be obtained from the organizations and Web sites listed in the Resources.

## Auditory-Oral

The Auditory-oral approach emphasizes maximum use of residual hearing through hearing aids or cochlear implants. Hearing is supplemented by visual cues (lipreading, facial expressions) but without the use of sign language.

## Auditory-Verbal

The Auditory-Verbal (AV) approach emphasizes hearing without using lipreading and other visual cues. Auditory stimulation is often provided in individual teaching sessions with the goal of preparing the child to function well in mainstream environments. In an Auditory-Verbal approach, the parent is regarded as the child's primary teacher.

## Cued Speech

Cued speech incorporates eight hand shapes (cues) representing different consonant sounds and places around the face representing the vowel sounds. "Cuing" provides a supplement to lipreading by making it easier for the child to differentiate sounds that look alike on the lips (such as /b/ and /p/).

## Total Communication

Total communication uses a combination of methods that include sign language, fingerspelling, and speechreading, in addition to hearing. Signing used with total communication follows English word order and grammar. Sign systems such as Signing Exact English take their core vocabulary from American Sign Language and combine it with signs created to represent the grammatical features of English.

## American Sign Language (Bilingual/Bicultural)

American Sign Language (ASL) is a manual language with its own grammatical rules, different from English and from sign systems that represent English. Those who advocate ASL as a first language for deaf children recommend that English be acquired as a *second* language, once a primary language base (via ASL) has been established.

## Communication Specialists

### Speech-Language Pathologist (SLP)

If your family chooses a spoken language approach, an SLP is likely to play an important role in helping your child learn to communicate orally. A qualified SLP will have a master's or doctoral degree from an accredited university program and will have experience using the communication approach the parent has chosen. In the United States, most SLP's will also be certified by the American Speech-Language-Hearing Association (ASHA) and licensed by the state. In Canada, certification with the Canadian Association of Speech-Language Pathologists and Audiologists (CASLPA) is optional for SLPs; certification is required to work at any institution accredited by CASLPA. In some Canadian provinces, and territories, the SLP must also have a license to practice.

Your child's SLP is someone with whom your family may well have a long relationship, so you'll want to make sure it's a healthy and happy one. One way to ensure that you're starting off right is to find a well qualified SLP. I knew even before Elizabeth saw an SLP for the first time that she had trouble pronouncing certain sounds—her /s/ sounded like /th/ and she mixed up her /p/ and /f/ sounds so that *put* came out as *foot*. Children with severe-to-profound hearing loss may not be producing *any* speech sounds clearly. Even for kids with normal hearing, certain speech sounds develop later than others (/r/, /l/, and /s/, for example), but in Elizabeth's case the problems may have been exacerbated by her hearing loss. Like most children who aren't diagnosed and fitted with hearing aids until relatively late, she hadn't heard all the sounds she needed to develop proper speech skills.

Historically, the more severe the hearing loss, the more severe the speech and language problems. But for children who have had the benefit of early diagnosis and appropriate hearing technology, the situation is changing. An SLP experienced at working with hard-of-hearing children can be helpful regardless of the degree of hearing loss. In addition to evaluating how a child produces speech sounds, the SLP will evaluate the receptive language ability—what the child understands. The SLP can also help your child develop auditory processing skills: learning to listen, recognize words, and make sense of what he's hearing. In normal-hearing children, this ability develops automatically.

If your child needs speech therapy, the SLP will develop a program to teach him to speak clearly and audibly. Developing age-appropriate speech and language skills takes time and work. Children with more severe hearing losses or with hearing loss combined with other challenges may require several sessions each week. A child with a milder loss may have only a few sessions a month. Either way, the SLP will give your child exercises to practice. Do them together whenever possible. If the exercises don't appear to be interesting to your child, ask the SLP for something different. If he isn't connecting with your child, either because of inexperience or a personality conflict, do your best to find a more suitable match. Other parents are often your best resource.

## Auditory-Verbal Therapist

As noted earlier, AV therapy emphasizes *listening* to develop spoken language and improve communication and social skills. It works well for children with all degrees of hearing loss who benefit from hearing aids and for children with profound hearing losses who benefit from cochlear implantation.

AV therapists and educators are certified by the Alexander Graham Bell Association for the Deaf and Hard of Hearing through its Academy for Listening and Spoken Language. Listening and Spoken Language specialists (LSLS) may be certified as auditory-verbal therapists (Cert AVT) or as auditory-verbal educators (Cert AVEd). According to the Alexander Graham Bell Academy Web site (see Resources), AV therapy is designed to optimize acquisition of spoken language through early diagnosis, one-on-one therapy, and state-of-the-art audiologic management and technology. An AV therapist, whose background may be in deaf education, speech pathology, or audiology often works one on one with a child. The therapist also works with the child's parents and caregivers, who play a key role by taking on the responsibility of implementing AV practice throughout the day. AV therapy is an ongoing process that may continue for months or even years.

## Signing Instructor

If you choose a manual system of communication, your child and your family will need to learn it. There are a number of manual systems, but the most common in North America are ASL and Signing Exact English (SEE). As noted earlier, ASL is a visual-spatial language separate from English. It has its own unique grammar, structure, and vocabulary. As with any new language, learning takes time and effort. ASL is used primarily by deaf people who do not use hearing aids or cochlear implants. SEE is a system that borrows its core signs from ASL, but adds signs so that English can be accurately represented on the hands. It, too, is primarily a manual form of communication. Because it follows the word order and rule features of English, it is easier for parents to learn. Some experts feel that the use of an English rule-based sign system facilitates the acquisition of English, whereas others feel that deaf children are better off acquiring a natural language, ASL, and then acquiring English as a second language. Families who favor the use of sign language and sign systems will find the National Association of the Deaf (NAD) a valuable resource (see Resources).

## Interpreter/Translator

If you choose to use sign language or a sign system, an interpreter, translator, or transliterator will translate a speaker's words into either ASL or a signing system such as SEE. Some hard-of-hearing children may need an oral interpreter or translator or transliterator in school or group activities.

The interpreter, translator, or transliterator must be fluent both in the spoken language being used and in the sign language or sign system your child uses. Otherwise, your child will not have access to all that is being said. The interpreter, translator, or transliterator will also translate what your child says into spoken English, so that your child can actively participate in discussions. This service provider should be well qualified and should not change the information or apply his own interpretation to what is being said or signed.

As with any profession, some interpreters, translators, and transliterators are better than others. If you choose to use a sign system, it's important to check your service provider's credentials and references to make sure he is qualified for the job. It's also important to check with your child and his teachers to make sure the service provider is performing his duties appropriately.

## Teacher of the Deaf and Hard of Hearing

In the past, most children with hearing loss were educated in special schools for the deaf. Nowadays most children with hearing loss are integrated into regular classrooms. Even those who require special instruction are likely to be served in regular schools. An itinerant teacher of the deaf and hard of hearing may work with your child outside the regular classroom and may also serve as a consultant to you and to school personnel. This person is likely to have a bachelor's or master's degree in special education and/or education of the deaf. Her responsibilities include making sure your child's educational needs are being met, which can mean working with teachers to help them understand your child's needs and equipment, helping with the transition between schools and with graduation from high school, making sure equipment is functioning and possibly making minor adjustments, monitoring your child's speech and language development, and providing one-on-one tutoring. Most itinerant teacher specialists are responsible for many students, so they travel from school to school and may work with your child for only an hour or two a week.

As parents, we don't expect to develop close friendships with the medical and audiology professionals who treat our children, though after years of checkups, exams, fitting, and repairs, it's not unusual for that to happen. The same may not hold true with the specialists who help guide our children through their school years, in part because we're not with our children throughout the school day. Still, I can't emphasize enough how important it is to develop a good working relationship with them, even once your child is out of elementary school. They may play a significant role in your child's education. For some parents, they will be a primary contact during the school years. As you'll discover while reading Chapter 9 and Chapter 10, working together with these nonmedical specialists is one of the best ways to help your child and to maximize the chances of making the school years enjoyable and productive.

# 4

# HEARING AIDS AND FM SYSTEMS

## The Modern Hearing Aid: Good Things Come in Small Packages

The first time I saw a child-sized hearing aid, I wanted to cry. It was about the size of one knuckle, yet it seemed enormous. I thought hearing aids were for senior citizens, not for a lively little girl with her whole life ahead of her.

When Elizabeth's audiologist, Paulette, said, "They're really quite small—years ago they were much bigger," I was convinced she was in deeper denial than I. "They look like the Empire State Building," I blurted out.

"Well, at least she has long hair," Paulette said in an unsuccessful attempt to make me feel better.

Nothing could have made me feel better. I hadn't yet reached the point where I was focusing on the reality that, unappealing though they were at the time, hearing aids were going to make things better for Elizabeth.

I'm not alone. It's hard enough for parents to accept that their child has a hearing loss, but at least until the child is aided we can continue to fool ourselves into believing nothing has changed, nothing is wrong. Once hearing aids become part of the picture, especially when they seem so massive and visible, denial becomes more difficult. However, for the vast majority of children, hearing aids improve everything from communication to behavior.

Many parents have asked their audiologist why their child can't have those nice little hearing aids that fit right inside the ears.

They're called in-the-ear (ITE) instruments. The tinier ones that are completely in the ear canal are called, not surprisingly, completely-in-the-canal (CIC) instruments. It's important to remember that the needs of a child differ from those of an adult, and that some features that may be helpful for adults may not be for children.

Neither ITE nor CIC instruments have the advantages that behind-the-ear (BTE) aids provide for children. BTE aids (Figure 4–1a and Figure 4–1b) are more versatile, they're compatible with other devices that will help your child, and they offer better control of whistling (which the experts refer to as *acoustic feedback*). Their size will also prove to be an advantage on those occasions, and let's hope they're rare, when your child loses them on the soccer field or the beach or the playroom floor.

Picking up Elizabeth at a birthday party when she was about 6 years old, I met a mom who has worn hearing aids since the mid-1960s, when she was 3. Paige noticed Elizabeth's aids almost immediately, perhaps because she was wearing one blue one and one red one, and at the time her earmolds had colored sparkles in them. (She's since gotten different colored aids and started wearing multi-

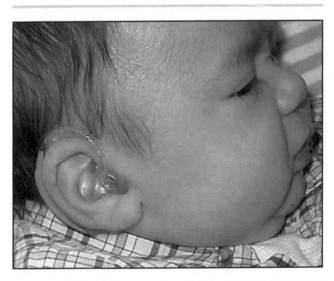

**Figure 4–1a.** An 8-week-old infant fitted with BTE hearing aids. Courtesy of Patricia Roush, University of North Carolina Hospitals.

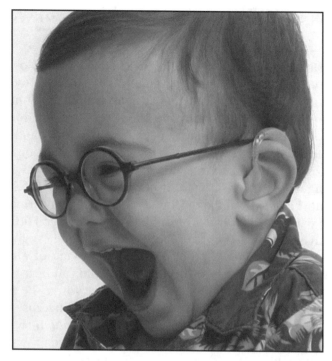

**Figure 4–1b.** A 3-year-old child fitted with BTE hearing aids. Courtesy of Patricia Roush, University of North Carolina School of Medicine.

colored molds.) "She's lucky," Paige said to me. "Hearing aids are so much better now than when I was a kid."

Indeed, hearing aids are a lot better now than they were as recently as the 1980s, and hearing aids from that era were a huge leap forward from the earliest versions. Hearing aids, in one form or another, have been around for centuries. The first attempts to amplify sound used animal horns and other devices fashioned into "ear trumpets." Early experiments with electricity resulted in the development of amplifiers that provided a greater increase in sound than nonelectric devices. In fact, Alexander Graham Bell, inventor of the telephone, was first a teacher of the deaf whose goal was to develop an electric hearing aid. But it wasn't until hearing aids moved from vacuum tubes to transistors in the second half of the 20th century that they became capable of delivering clear amplified sounds.

# How Hearing Aids (Are Supposed to) Work

The hearing aids of today are technological marvels employing tiny sophisticated components and circuitry. For parents they can be puzzling and even a bit overwhelming, at least in the beginning. The main purpose of a hearing aid is to make speech and environmental sounds audible without exceeding levels of comfortable listening. Your child's audiologist will refer to the latter phenomenon as *loudness discomfort*. As noted earlier, the most practical option for infants and young children is a BTE aid, also known as an ear-level aid.

In most cases the audiologist will recommend a hearing aid for each ear, which is known as a binaural fitting. A binaural fitting may not be advisable if a child has useable hearing in one ear and a profound hearing loss in the other ear. The advantage of a binaural fitting is that with both ears working, your child can hear better in a noisy environment and more easily determine where the sound is coming from (this is known as *sound localization*). Because hearing aid microphones can be located at ear level, *stereophonic* reception can be achieved, as well as an increase in high-frequency amplification. Another advantage of a binaural fitting is that your child is always likely to have at least one functional hearing aid in the event of a malfunction, although it's always best if your audiologist can provide a loaner hearing aid at those times. Finally, BTE hearing aids can also be "coupled to" FM systems, discussed later in this chapter.

A hearing aid has several components. The microphone picks up incoming sound waves and converts them to electrical signals. The amplifier increases the intensity and, when necessary, further modifies the incoming sound. The receiver converts electrical signals back to sound waves that are delivered, through the earmold, to the ear of the listener.

Modern hearing aids use digital technology. The simplest way to understand what digital means is to think about a clock. Clocks traditionally used continuous movement of gears and hands to display information regarding the hour and minute. Digital clocks, instead of providing a continuous stream, divide the hour into segments that are displayed as numbers. Attached to a computer, a digital hearing aid can be programmed by the audiologist to provide the appropriate amount of amplification across a range frequencies where audibility is needed to hear speech and environmental sounds.

Other features, such as noise and feedback control and various circuit designs, can also be implemented.

One of the circuit designs favored by many pediatric audiologists is called *wide dynamic range compression* (WDRC). Although this sounds highly technical (and it is), the purpose of WDRC and why many audiologists prefer it for children is simple: hearing aids with WDRC are designed to take soft sounds and make them louder, and to take very loud sounds and make them softer. Because children are subjected to listening environments that cover a wide range of sound levels, WDRC helps them hear comfortably as conditions change. Another important feature is the microphone design. A *directional mic* amplifies sounds in front of the listener more than sounds at the side or behind the listener. In contrast, *omnidirectional* mics surround the listener in a more natural way. For infants and young children most audiologists will recommend omnidirectional mics, but as your child gets older there may be situations where directional mics will be helpful. Your audiologist will explain how these microphones work and which is most appropriate for your child.

Remote controls for hearing aids can also be helpful, allowing parents to turn a device on or off or to activate/deactivate directional microphones without interrupting the child's activities. By 7 or 8 years of age most children can take responsibility for these adjustments. Some newer hearing aids also have a remote device designed to check the functionality, including the volume and program settings and remaining battery life. This can be especially useful for monitoring hearing aid function in very young children.

## The Earmold: A Blessing and a Curse

I was still in shock about Elizabeth's diagnosis the first time I heard the term *earmold*. Had I been in a better mood I probably would have laughed out loud. Let's face it, it's a pretty odd-sounding term for something that is critical to your child's hearing.

Earmolds for children are made of a soft, compliant material. Some children are allergic to the standard materials and this will become apparent if your child develops a rash or swelling. Fortunately, special hypoallergenic materials are available when needed.

In any event, the process of making an earmold is the same. The audiologist inserts into your child's ear canal a cotton or foam ball with a string attached. Using a plastic syringe, the audiologist will then fill the canal with soft silicone to make a form, also known as an impression, which will be sent to a laboratory where it will be made into a custom mold, perfectly fitted (we hope) to your child's ear. Within the earmold is a clear plastic tube that connects the earmold to the BTE hearing aid.

It sounds simple, but early earmold experiences can be terrifying for your child. I know they were for Elizabeth—and for me. For her, it was the idea of having her ear filled with gunk for what seemed like ages (though in truth it took only a few minutes). For me it was fear that the string would break and the silicone would be lodged in her ear forever. Both our fears were groundless. In fact, Elizabeth now looks forward to having earmolds made because the audiologist always lets her play with the little bits of extra silicone, which are like modeling clay, until they dry, at which point they become smooth and even a bit bouncy.

Elizabeth's first earmolds seemed to fit very snugly into her ears—so snugly, in fact, that I often had a difficult time putting them in. I eventually discovered that swabbing them with a diaper wipe just before inserting them provided the right amount of lubrication. A better solution is a lubricant called Otoease (Figure 4–2), or similar products which you can get from your audiologist. As Elizabeth grew, her earmolds slipped in more easily. As I became a more experienced mother of a hard-of-hearing child, I learned that when putting in the earmolds was too easy, they were probably too small and it was time for new ones. The greater the hearing loss, the more critical it is for the earmolds to fit snugly.

## Selecting and Fitting the Hearing Aid: What Your Audiologist Will Do

Before the hearing aids can be fitted, the audiologist needs to determine how much hearing loss there is and how the hearing sensitivity differs across the frequency range for each ear. For example, a child whose loss is only in the high frequencies (a *high-frequency* hear-

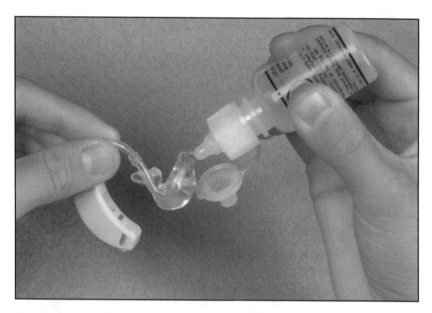

**Figure 4–2.** Otoease, a lubricant, is applied to an earmold to make insertion easier.

ing loss) needs different amplification from one whose hearing loss is about the same in all frequencies (a *flat* hearing loss).

Infants cannot be evaluated using behavioral tests until they reach a developmental age of about 6 months. Therefore, their hearing levels must be determined using physiologic tests. Recall from Chapter 3 that diagnostic auditory brainstem responses (ABR), which can be obtained from a sleeping baby, are needed to provide an estimate of hearing sensitivity across a range of frequencies.

Once there is sufficient information to determine the degree of hearing loss and the amount of loss across a range of frequencies, your audiologist will decide the most appropriate type of hearing aids and how they should be adjusted. To do this she'll use special instruments designed to measure the amplification in each frequency region.

*Real-ear measures* involve placing a microphone in the ear canal to accurately determine the amount of amplification delivered to the ear. Accurate measurements are critical because infants have smaller ears than older children or adults. Even within an age group there may be differences in the size, shape, and other ear characteristics. The most important difference is the smaller size of the ear canal. Because of the way sound levels are affected by the amount of space between the tip of the earmold and the eardrum, infants get more amplification than older children even when the same hearing aid is adjusted to the same settings. Think of it in terms of noise levels in a room: If you play a stereo at full blast in an auditorium, the volume level may be just right. But play it at full blast in a small room and the noise will be overwhelming.

Figure 4-3 shows probe microphone measurements being obtained in the ear canal of a 3-month-old. In addition to checking the amplification levels for typical sounds such as speech, it's also important to check the hearing aid's maximum output to ensure that the hearing aid does not exceed safe and comfortable listening

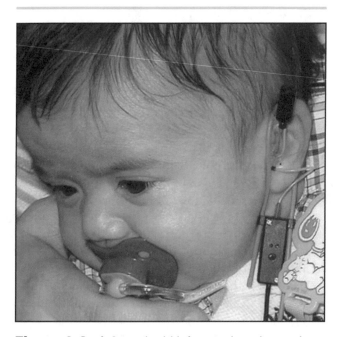

**Figure 4–3.** A 6-week-old infant undergoing real-ear measures for initial hearing aid fitting. Courtesy of Patricia Roush, University of North Carolina School of Medicine.

levels. In fact, excessive amplification can cause a child to reject hearing aids. In extreme cases, overamplification can even damage the cochlea. However, an overly conservative approach results in amplification levels that are too low, providing little or no aided benefit.

In recent years audiologists have developed an alternative strategy that reduces the amount of time the child is required to have the probe microphone in the ear. Calculating *real ear to coupler differences* (RECD) results in greater ease of testing.

## How Much Benefit Should You Expect?

Many people think hearing aids are like eyeglasses: wear them and everything comes in clearly. That's not the case. True, hearing aids have improved technologically in recent years, and some are even becoming fashionable (instead of being limited to flesh-colored cases and clear earmolds, there is now a rainbow of colors from which to choose). But although hearing aids boost the intensity of sound and perform other enhancements, they cannot fully compensate for the lack of clarity that often occurs with a sensorineural hearing loss. Also, it needs to be understood that the greater the hearing loss, the harder the hearing aids have to work. Even when using hearing aids, a person with a severe-to-profound hearing loss is not likely to hear as well as someone with a mild-to-moderate loss. Parents can play an important role in monitoring and recording their child's progress with amplification. Two functional assessment tools developed for parents by audiologist Karen Anderson are the Early Language Function (ELF) and the Child Home Inventory of Listening Difficulties (CHILD; see Resources). These parent inventories allow family members and caretakers to monitor their child's progress and better understand the implications of hearing loss.

## How Long Do Hearing Aids Last?

As with any electronic device, parts eventually break or wear out. Your child's audiologist should be able to help you determine when it's time to purchase new instruments. Hearing aids are expensive.

Be sure to consult with your audiologist regarding purchase options and, in some cases, programs to assist with purchase. Because of technological advances your child will likely hear differently with her new aids, which will probably be more sophisticated than her last pair. It's a good idea to have your audiologist tell your child, in advance, to expect some changes in how she hears. In most cases she will adapt quickly and like them even better than the old ones.

## Bone Conduction Hearing Aid

Most permanent hearing losses in children are due to abnormal *inner ear* function (i.e., sensorineural impairment). There are rare congenital conditions, however, that result in a hearing loss due to middle and/or outer ear abnormalities. These losses are often associated with normal inner ear function. When an outer ear problem makes it impossible to use a standard earmold and hearing aid, a *bone conduction* device may be recommended. The sound is delivered using vibrations directly to the inner ear by a bone vibrator worn on the head. Although a bit cumbersome, this arrangement can provide the stimulation necessary to help a child acquire language and develop speech. Some parents cleverly adapt hats or headbands for this purpose. When children are around 7 or 8 and the bones in their skull have sufficient density, they can be considered for a bone-anchored hearing aid (BAHA), a surgically implanted device coupled to the head by way of a titanium screw.

## FM Systems

Most of us would be lost without our local FM radio stations, but we rarely think about how the signals get to us. Somewhere there's a transmitter where the sound begins. The signals are then delivered to an antenna, often a high tower on a hillside where electromagnetic waves (not sound waves) are transmitted to FM radios in homes, cars, and buildings. In other words, FM transmission requires a sound source, a transmitter, an antenna, and a receiver.

The FM devices used with hearing aids work on the same basic principles. Their components include a microphone, a transmitter (with an antenna) connected to the microphone, and an FM receiver. The person talking—a parent, teacher, coach, or scout leader—wears the microphone/transmitter (Figure 4-4) and the child wears the receiver (Figure 4-5) coupled to her hearing aids or cochlear implant. The microphone may be worn around the neck, on a headband, or clipped to a piece of clothing, but the best option in most cases is a small "boom mic" like the ones used for hands-free use of a cell phone.

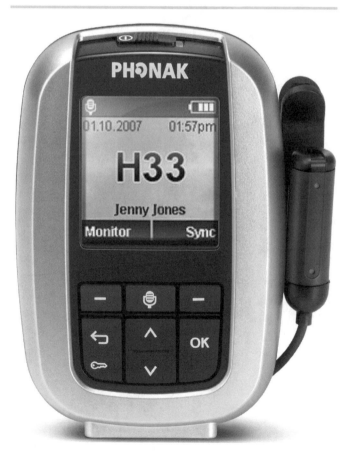

**Figure 4–4.** FM transmitter. Courtesy of Phonak.

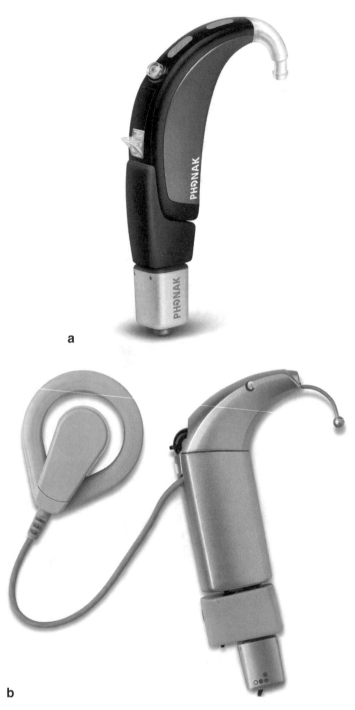

a

b

**Figure 4–5.** FM receiver attached to a BTE hearing aid (**a**) and cochlear implant (**b**). Courtesy of Phonak.

The transmission range, although far less than the local FM station, is more than adequate for most listening situations. The advantage of an FM system is that amplified sounds are delivered to the ear as if the person speaking were only a few inches from the person talking. In other words, regardless of the distance between the speaker and listener, signals arriving at the ear are the same as if the child were close to the person talking. A potential disadvantage is that if anyone else is talking at the same time as the primary speaker (the person controlling the microphone), the child will have trouble hearing other voices. This problem is overcome by adjusting the hearing to deliver FM only (when appropriate) or FM plus hearing aid (with the hearing aid at a level slightly lower than FM). Other sound sources, such as the audio signal from a TV or video recorder, can also be delivered via FM. The most important advantage of FM is that the listener receives the signal at a level well above the background noise. The outcome is an improvement in the level of the primary signal (your voice, for example) in comparison to competing background noise.

Audiologists sometimes use the term *signal-to-noise ratio* to express the relationship between speech and noise. When the signal-to-noise-ratio is 0 it means that the primary signal and the background noise are at equal levels. Unfortunately, people with hearing loss are often required to communicate in situations where the background noise level is as high as or even higher than the primary signal. This is regrettable considering that research has clearly shown that people with hearing loss require a *better* listening environment than people with normal hearing to achieve the same level of understanding. Although FM cannot create a perfect listening environment, it can greatly reduce the problems of background noise, speaker-listener distance, and reverberation (echo), all factors known to make listening more difficult.

Several options are available for getting the FM signal to the child's ear, but it's important to remember that she needs to hear her own voice as well as the sound delivered by the FM transmitter. This is accomplished by combining the amplified sound provided by the hearing aid with the FM signal. Several options are available for receiving the FM signal (Figure 4–6). Fully dedicated FM receivers are relatively small and sleek in appearance but they lack versatility; that is, if there's a change in hearing aids, the dedicated FM receiver will not be interchangeable. Universal FM receivers, although

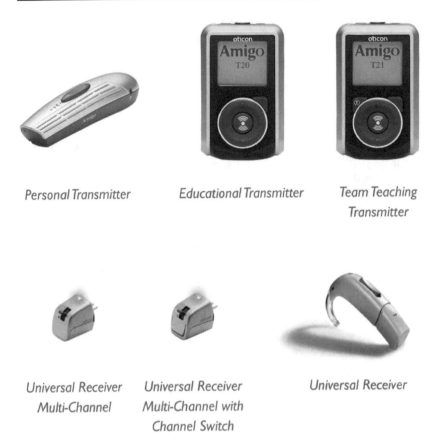

Personal Transmitter    Educational Transmitter    Team Teaching
Transmitter

Universal Receiver    Universal Receiver    Universal Receiver
Multi-Channel    Multi-Channel with
Channel Switch

**Figure 4–6.** FM transmitters and receivers in a variety of configurations. Courtesy of Oticon.

slightly larger, can be used with many different brands of hearing aids and thus offer greater flexibility. Fully integrated FM receivers are the smallest because they are built into the design of the hearing aid, but when considering this option it's important to make sure that the hearing aid has all the features and adjustment capabilities your child needs. Your audiologist will recommend the best option for your child.

In most listening situations the hearing aid microphone must be activated to allow the child to hear her own speech as well as the speech of others in the immediate vicinity. In other situations, where only the input from the FM is important (for example when listening to an audio recording), the hearing aid microphone can be switched off. Proper location and use of the microphone are critical. That is, the FM microphone/transmitter must be located near the source of the primary input signal (teacher's or parent's mouth, another child or sibling, television, tape player, and so on) in order to get the full advantage of FM. To eliminate amplifying unwanted environmental sounds, special audio input cables are available to allow direct transmission of devices such as computers, iPods, and TV to the hearing instruments. It is important for parents, caretakers, and teachers to understand proper use of FM because an inappropriately used system can create a poorer listening situation than hearing aids used alone.

The signals sent by FM systems travel on specific frequencies. The frequency of the transmitter and receiver must be compatible. It is important to be aware of interactions between devices. I once heard about a girl who spent the first half of the academic year convinced she was going crazy because whenever she was in school, she heard voices. In French. She was embarrassed to tell her mother what was going on inside her head. What she didn't realize at the time was that she wasn't the only hard-of-hearing child in the school. Unbeknownst to her, a student in the French immersion program was also using an FM, and he was on the same channel. Once the FMs were put on different channels, the problem was solved. Some school districts have access to an educational audiologist to assist in sorting out these issues. If an audiologist is not involved in the management of classroom listening equipment, you may want to advocate for this (see Chapter 9).

Don't be surprised if your child eventually says she doesn't want to use the FM system. Usually around the time they reach junior high school, kids become increasingly determined to blend in with everyone else. The mother of a middle-schooler told me her daughter's protest went like this: "When I get married do you think my husband's going to use the FM during the wedding ceremony?"

Toby wanted to quit using his FM in sixth grade, but his mother wouldn't let him. He's grateful for that. "You don't miss anything the teacher says," he points out. By 11th grade, though, he abandoned it altogether. Although he has a moderate-to-severe loss, if there was no background noise in class he could hear well enough to get by, and he was finding it more trouble than it was worth.

"It was this thing I had to truck around with me all the time and it wasn't benefiting me as much," he says, adding that going without forced him to pay attention. "I just sat at the front of the room and told myself, 'I'm not going to have this when I get out of here, so I might as well get used to it.'"

Fortunately, this scenario is changing: assistive listening devices are increasingly common not just in school settings, but in the wider world. FM, infrared, and other technologies are available in theaters, auditoriums, and places of worship. In the United States, the Americans with Disabilities Act (ADA) ensures that communication is accessible to people with hearing loss, just as a building is accessible to people with physical disabilities. Moreover, people with hearing loss are incorporating assistive listening devices into their daily lives to enhance communication with friends, family members, and coworkers. I was warned that Elizabeth wouldn't want to use her FM in school by the time she reached seventh grade, and the warnings proved true. But whenever she's on an airplane, it's one of the first things she pulls from her backpack, because it's the only way she can listen to the movie. She plugs the FM cord into the armrest where the headphones normally go and she's ready to enjoy the in-flight entertainment.

With the popularity of MP3 players and cell phones, hearing aids and assistive listening devices are not as noticeable or stigmatizing as they once were. Eventually our children will become their own advocates. For now, we must encourage them to take advantage of available accommodations to the listening environment through technology and by educating those with normal hearing.

## Sound Field FM

The sound field listening system is an example of FM technology that is sometimes used in a classroom setting with older children who have milder hearing losses. In this arrangement, a teacher wears a microphone/transmitter and the FM signal is transmitted to a receiver/amplifier. The signal is broadcast through loudspeakers, enabling the teacher to move freely around the room. Because a microphone is worn close to the teacher's mouth, amplified signals are heard at consistent levels throughout the classroom.

Although this arrangement is not as good as personal FM, it is a less expensive option that has the advantage of providing a more favorable listening environment, even for normal-hearing classmates.

A final consideration is Bluetooth, the technology that allows wireless electronic devices to communicate with each other. The wireless link is made possible by radio waves that connect Bluetooth-compatible devices over a short range, usually within 30 feet. This technology has been in use for several years but is now becoming more standardized and better suited for use with hearing aids. There are two main advantages. First, Bluetooth enables a listener's binaural hearing aids to communicate with each other in ways that provide better amplification and "stereophonic" reception. The second is that Bluetooth allows hearing aids to connect to other wireless devices such as cell phones, MP3 players, and personal computers. Most of the hearing aid companies have introduced Bluetooth compatible hearing instruments. Your audiologist can tell you more about this technology and whether it would be appropriate for your child.

## What If the Hearing Loss Is Only in One Ear?

*A* unilateral *hearing loss is one that affects only one ear. People with unilateral hearing loss often have difficulty determining the location of a sound or understanding speech in a noisy situation, especially when sounds are directed toward the nonhearing or poorer-hearing ear.*

*Diagnosis requires medical assessment by an ear specialist (ENT) to determine if the loss is medically treatable and whether it might be associated with other conditions. The diagnosis may require imaging or other tests. Assessment by an audiologist is necessary to determine the amount and type of hearing loss, and if a hearing aid or other hearing technology is recommended. When a unilateral sensorineural loss is in the mild-moderate range, some children may benefit from a* monaural *hearing aid fitting, especially if the loss is detected early. In cases of more severe unilateral hearing loss, amplifying the abnormal ear may be detrimental to the child's overall hearing. The audiologist will help make this determination.*

*Most children with unilateral hearing loss do well in school, but studies have shown that as many as one third are at risk for educational problems. Careful monitoring of the child's hearing and listening environment is essential. Limiting background noise whenever possible is especially important. An FM system may be helpful. The child with unilateral hearing loss should be aware of the need for extra care around traffic and other hazardous situations.*

# 5

# COCHLEAR IMPLANTS

One of the first questions friends and relatives asked after they learned about Elizabeth's hearing loss was whether she was going to get a cochlear implant. The answer was no, it was never a consideration. Elizabeth has enough residual hearing to use hearing aids successfully. That's because her cochleas and auditory nerves have enough function to benefit from the amplified sound that hearing aids provide. But for children and adults whose residual hearing is severely limited, cochlear implants have made an important and, in many ways, astounding difference: they allow deaf people to hear.

"I cannot say how much it has changed my life for the better," says Jenny, 24, who is profoundly deaf and received a cochlear implant at age 16. Until then, she had worn hearing aids since she was 8 months old. "Before the implant I was shy and withdrawn," she says. "I was insecure about myself, usually due to my hearing loss, as I could not speak very well or understand people easily. Since the implant, my speech has improved tremendously. I can understand people a lot more easily. My fear of speaking to strangers has faded. Nowadays I can chat with a complete stranger with confidence, all thanks to the cochlear implant."

Cochlear implants were first used in the late 1970s, but those devices were not nearly as sophisticated as the ones that Jenny and others use today. People with the first generation of implants could hear, but they weren't able to easily distinguish what they were hearing; at best, implants provided sound awareness and an aid to lipreading. Consequently, the best candidates for early implants were adults who had lost their hearing late in life, after having acquired normal speech and language; they remembered what things sounded like. Children who received implants were often well into adolescence and far less likely to hear well, much less develop appropriate speech and language skills. Today and since 2002, the Food and Drug Administration (FDA), which monitors the use of medical prosthetics in the United States, has approved cochlear implants for use in children 12 months of age and older. Guidelines are similar in Canada. On occasion, a child will receive an implant before turning 1, but this is considered an "off-label" use of the device. Research is underway to determine the risk and benefits of providing an implant before 12 months. It is well documented that congenitally deaf children who receive cochlear implants at 12 months, and have appropriate therapy, can overcome the effects of auditory deprivation during the first year of life and attain language milestones typical of their hearing peers.

## What Is a Cochlear Implant?

To understand cochlear implants it's important to remember how the ear works. As I explained in Chapter 2, the ear is divided into three parts: the outer ear, the middle ear, and the inner ear. Sound waves traveling down the ear canal cause the eardrum to move, which makes the bones of the middle ear vibrate. Those vibrations stimulate the hair cells of the cochlea, a pea-sized, spiral-shaped organ deep in the inner ear. The cochlea sends signals to the auditory nerve that are transmitted to the brain, where sounds are interpreted.

Most cochlear implant candidates have normal outer and middle ear function. But when their inner ear fluids are stimulated, the hair cells of the cochlea do not respond or have such a limited response that signals reaching the brain provide minimal information. People who benefit from hearing aids have enough. For them, hearing aids help by amplifying incoming sounds.

A cochlear implant provides a detour around the hair cells. The implant contains a number of parts, including an array of electrodes implanted in the cochlea. Those electrodes stimulate the auditory nerve fibers directly, from *within* the inner ear. As shown in Figure 5-1, incoming sounds are picked up by a microphone, which delivers them to a speech processor; a small computer analyzes the incoming sounds and converts them to an electrical code. The coded electrical signals travel from the speech processor to a transmitting coil, across the skin, to an implanted receiver where the electrical signals are delivered from the auditory nerve to the brain.

The first generation of implants was capable of delivering only a limited amount of auditory information. Current models have multiple channels and electrodes that allow users to perceive a much broader range and complexity of sounds, including speech.

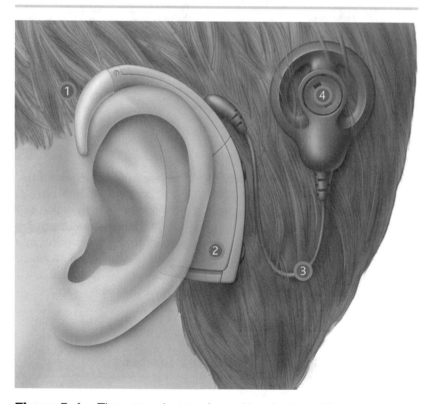

**Figure 5–1a.** The external parts of a cochlear implant. (1) retention hook, (2) speech processor, (3) cable connector, (4) radio transmitting coil.

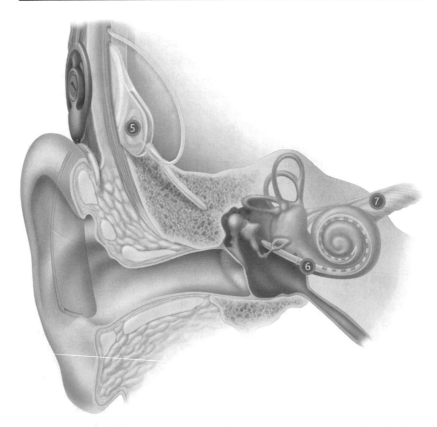

**Figure 5–1b.** The internal parts of a cochlear implant. (5) radio frequency receiver, (6) electrode array, (7) auditory nerve (not part of implant). The sound processor converts incoming sounds to digital signals that are transmitted across the skin to the internal receiver. The internal receiver then routes the digital signals to the electrode array where electrical impulses bypass the damaged hair cells and stimulate the auditory nerve. From there the nerve impulses travel to the brain where they are perceived as sound. Courtesy of Cochlear Corporation.

## Cochlear Implant Surgery

Cochlear implant surgery is performed under general anesthesia. An otologist (ear surgeon) performs the surgery, making an incision behind the ear to expose the skull. A small area on the bone is then hollowed slightly to make room for the internal receiver. The surgeon then drills through the bone to get access to the inner ear. Once the inner ear is opened the electrodes are inserted into the cochlea. The receiver is then secured onto the bone and stitches are used to close the incision. Most cochlear implant surgeries are uncomplicated and patients are usually able to go home the same day after a recovery period. After about two weeks the stitches are removed and the person can resume normal activities. There is usually a delay of about one month before the audiologist first activates the cochlear implant's external processor. The delay allows the incision to thoroughly heal.

## Risks of Cochlear Implantation

All surgical procedures involving general anesthesia carry some risks. There is also the risk of infection near the surgical site. Because there is also an increased risk of meningitis, immunizations must be up to date. Cochlear implant surgery, because it is performed near the facial nerve, also carries the risk of temporary or permanent damage to the nerve that controls facial feeling and movement. Some patients may report temporary changes in taste. All of these complications are very rare. If your child is being considered for cochlear implantation the otologist will go over the risks in detail. Most patients do experience some tenderness for a few days at the surgical site. Although it is sometimes possible to preserve hearing at pre-surgical levels, it is important to understand that in most cases some or all of the remaining residual hearing in the implanted ear will be lost when the implant is inserted. That's the reason implants are not considered for people who have enough residual hearing to use hearing aids successfully. The otologist and audiologist will advise you of risks and benefits.

## Who Is a Candidate and Which Device Is Best?

Deciding who is a cochlear implant candidate requires a team approach. Along with the parents, team members often include the otologist, audiologist, speech-language pathologist, educators of the deaf, and sometimes a psychologist or social worker. The process of evaluating a candidate includes assessing the child's use of residual hearing and potential for benefiting from hearing aids, as well as counseling the family. Parents or guardians making this important decision need to understand that it will affect their child's entire life. There will be costs of time, energy and resources. The potential benefits can be life changing but to obtain the maximum benefits, which must be weighed in relation to the risks of surgery, the family must understand the process and be committed to supporting their child. This includes maintaining hardware, advocating for therapeutic and educational services, and providing a home environment that nurtures the development of auditory skills of a two year old. (Figure 5–2).

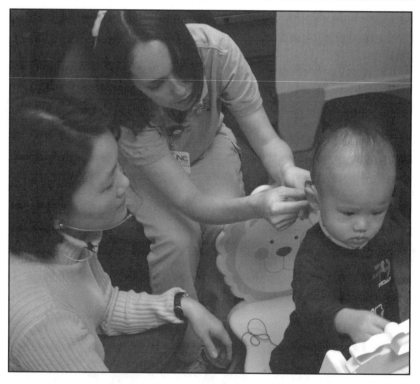

**Figure 5–2.** A cochlear implant is activated for the first time in a two year old child as his mother looks on. Courtesy of Kathryn Wilson, University of North Carolina School of Medicine.

Parents are sometimes surprised to learn that there are only a few manufacturers of cochlear implants in the world. In North America options include Cochlear Corporation, based in Australia; Advanced Bionics, based in California; and Med-El, based in Austria. All three devices are well-regarded and all three companies have good technical support in the US and Canada (see Resources for websites and additional information). Not all cochlear implant centers offer all three implant systems. The cochlear implant team will counsel families about their options.

If your child is a cochlear implant candidate you may wonder which of the three manufacturers is best. The implant team will provide information about various options. In some cases the team may feel that a particular device is better suited for the specific needs of your child.

When considering cochlear implantation it's always a good idea to talk with other parents. That's what Deborah and Jerry did when their daughter, Riley, became a potential implant candidate shortly before her second birthday in 2000. The family support group they belonged to had children with cochlear implants, so they had a sense of how the devices worked. They got more information while attending an Auditory Verbal conference, where the three cochlear implant manufacturers had sent representatives. The couple went armed with a list of questions, all of which were answered satisfactorily. But ultimately they relied less on company representatives than on their impressions of implanted children, particularly their speech and language skills, and conversations with the parents of those children.

"All the companies were very helpful but ultimately the best and most helpful information came from the parents," says Deborah, who is confident that she and her husband made the right choice for Riley. Their daughter is an independent elementary school student who loves dancing, cooking, reading, and running. Riley also takes Chinese and Hebrew classes after school and on weekends. "You couldn't pick her out of the whole grade as being deaf," Deborah says.

That's the way it is with many children today who receive cochlear implants at an early age. Dr. Craig Buchman, an ear surgeon at the University of North Carolina at Chapel Hill, who has performed hundreds of implant surgeries, says that all of the major cochlear implant manufacturers produce devices that are highly effective for improving auditory abilities. "You'd be hard-pressed to show an objective difference in performance among the currently available devices," he explains. "Device choice is probably more often about what appeals to the patient or the family, as well as the reliability of the device, rather than which one performs better."

## What Happens after Cochlear Implantation?

Once the cochlear implant is activated it requires a careful adjustment period called "mapping," which involves programming the implant's speech processor for optimal hearing. Proper mapping also ensures that speech and environmental sounds will not exceed levels of comfortable listening. The mapping is done by an audiologist who specializes in cochlear implants and who will adjust the device to create a sound or speech coding program based on your child's response to electrical stimulation. The mapping process typically requires frequent visits at the beginning and may continue over a period of months. For optimal use and benefit, the hardware must be well maintained and your child will need semi-annual check-ups, depending on age and use. Changes occur as the child becomes more accustomed to sound and as more information is acquired about his use of the device.

Jenny remembers everything about her first mapping session, which took place when she was 16. "The minute the audiologist turned on my implant for the first time was a huge breakthrough in my life," she says. "I remember she had silenced the fan that was on in the room before turning it on. She knew that the hum of the fan would probably startle me because I was not able to pick up that sound with hearing aids. When she turned on the implant I heard the loudest humming ever—it was almost overwhelming. It sounded like a jet airplane to my ears. It turns out that the roaring sound was the hum from the computer."

Today, eight years later, Jenny can barely hear a computer humming—but it's not because her hearing has gotten worse. Far from it. "I find that my hearing and speech keep improving every year," she says. "I have an easier time associating sound. In the beginning, if I heard an unfamiliar sound, I would have a hard time figuring out what it was."

For instance, she says, she can now tell the difference between a car engine and that of a lawnmower or a snowmobile. "However," she adds, "I still have lots of work to do in that area—I am always discovering new sounds."

## New Developments in Cochlear Implantation

As cochlear implants have improved so have the benefits. Much has been learned about the technology as well as the aspects of intervention. Research is ongoing and there is still much to learn but studies have shown that implants allow many children to make excellent progress with speech and language. As a result, implantation is being considered for a growing number of children even when there is residual hearing. The decision must be made carefully since implantation means the ear will no longer be able to receive sound in the usual manner. For this reason the implant team will often recommend implanting the poorer ear if there's a difference between the two. This allows a person to continue to use a hearing aid in one ear and a cochlear implant on the other.

Hailey has been using an implant and a hearing aid since she turned four in 2004. Diagnosed shortly after birth with a severe-to-profound loss in her right ear and a moderately-severe to severe loss in her left, Hailey had done very well with her hearing aids, but by the time she was ready for kindergarten her language skills were reaching a plateau and the hearing in her better ear was declining. The family was no stranger to implants: Hailey's brother, Carter, who is two years older, had been using an implant successfully since he was 19 months old. But using a hearing aid in one ear and an implant in the other was different, and Hailey didn't like it at first.

"She had to learn to integrate the signals from the implant with the signals from her hearing aid," recalls her mother, Cheri. "We had to stay on her to keep the implant on, but then she got to where she was fine with it. It's helped her out tremendously. Her speech is beautiful. She can carry on great conversations with the implant alone, with two of them together, or with hearing aid alone. In the morning she'll put on her hearing aid first, then chill out a bit, then put the implant on. I think she likes the hearing aid. There's a big difference when she doesn't have her implant on."

Listening through a hearing aid or a cochlear implant is a unique experience for every person. Much depends on the person's previous experience with sound, the level of language development and the length of device use. For Jenny, listening through a hearing aid is "worlds apart" from listening through an implant. According to her, "hearing aids amplify the surrounding sound around you, so in that context, it's my belief that you are hearing what the sound is actually supposed to sound like, frequency- and pitch-wise, but with a much, much lower intensity."

With the implant, she says, the pitches and frequencies are "artificially created" and as a result, "everything sounds a bit robotic, almost like the automated voices you hear from computers. Not that I mind at all!" she adds quickly. "It's certainly better than what I was hearing before. The computer in the implant is deadly accurate in picking up the pitches and frequencies. Everything is sharper, the sentences almost clippy, versus the monotonous drone I was hearing from hearing aids. I can hear the high frequency sounds such as "shh" so well. It's so sharp, which I love, because it has helped me with hearing and speaking."

Jenny is adept at describing her experiences because she has the language and experience to compare a hearing aid and a cochlear implant. Very young children who receive cochlear implants develop communication abilities based on a level of hearing that is uniquely "normal" for that individual. Not everyone achieves a similar level of performance, due to a number of factors, among them age at implant, status of the cochlea and higher auditory processing centers, therapeutic and educational support, and the presence of other medical, developmental, behavioral and cognitive conditions. Even if the person does not use a hearing aid, practical considerations and cost mean that cochlear implants are usually provided on one side only.

The standard of care has been to provide one cochlear implant for a child with bilateral hearing loss; however, many parents are opting for two. Studies of children with unilateral hearing loss indicate that some struggle educationally and socially compared to children with two normal-hearing ears. Not all insurance companies provide coverage for two implants, however, and many children have done well with just one. Bilateral implantation is a topic of much discussion at this time; policies and practices are under review and likely to undergo further change as more research evidence becomes available.

## Cochlear Implant Maintenance

As with hearing aids, cochlear implants are intended for full-time use. Therefore, they require ongoing maintenance. It's a good idea to have a dryer to store the external device when your child isn't using it, and back-up parts for components that are the most vulnerable, such as cables. Implants use rechargeable or standard disposable batteries and it's helpful to have several on hand.

"After we've had them for six to eight months and I recharge them, even a full battery won't last all day long," says Sharon, whose daughter, Regan, nine, received her first implant at 22 months and her second the summer between first and second grade.

"They wear down after a while—and if they go through the washer, they wear down a little sooner," jokes Sharon, who keeps up to six extra batteries at home. "I'm probably buying more batteries than other people," she acknowledges. Regan also keeps a charger in her classroom, with an extra battery.

Despite the best efforts, breakdowns occur. Parents, teachers, and other caretakers play a critical role in checking the external device and its cords, insuring that controls are at the proper settings, and making minor repairs when necessary. Hailey's brother, Carter, had been implanted a year when, at a routine exam, his audiologist discovered that the implant was failing.

"It made me realize how much we depended on that implant," Cheri recalls. "I remember taking him down to X-Ray to see if it was broken, and I had to tap him on the shoulder to communicate with him. Prior to that day, I could have taken him down there and said, 'Carter, come here,' and he would do what I told him. It was very humbling—it made me really appreciate what we have, although every night when we take it off, I realize we don't just take it for granted."

Just like getting a first cochlear implant is a difficult and personal decision for families, having a revision surgery or a second implant also requires contemplation and careful consideration. The first time Cheri suggested bilateral implantation to Carter around the time he was eight years old, he said no. He'd already undergone two surgeries to replace the initial implant, the first time when it failed and the second when he fell on the playground and damaged it. Cheri figured he didn't want to go through yet another surgery. But when she proposed the possibility again two years later, shortly after his tenth birthday, he said yes.

"He was starting to have a hard time in school and he didn't seem to be hearing as well," she says. "I'd also observed that it was harder to talk to him in real-life noisy situations."

Carter's audiologist and the team at UNC agreed that he was a good candidate. In the summer of 2008, Carter received an implant in his other ear. Within a week of having the implant activated, he was able to hear actual sounds instead of beeps, and he could tell his mother the number of syllables in words. He was also beginning to understand some words.

"It will be a slow process to get the new ear up to speed, but we're working as hard as we can," Cheri says. "We're keeping our fingers crossed that this will help Carter."

## How Much Do Cochlear Implants Cost and Who Pays?

Cochlear implants are expensive. Hardware and surgical fees cost thousands of dollars. The typical cost for the device and surgery is currently $40,000 to $60,000. Ongoing audiological care and rehabilitative services will also be needed. Maintenance needs are ongoing. Although all three companies offer a 10-year warranty on the internal device and a three-year warranty on the external components, planning for a life-time of maintenance costs cannot be overlooked. Upgrades in the technology also come at a cost. Additionally, the costs of habilitation may need to be considered. Not all school systems offer the kind of support a child needs. Private therapy may need to be arranged, at some cost. Fortunately, financial assistance is often available. It is important to thoroughly investigate insurance benefits available through your private insurance, or assistance available through state or provincial agencies. The cochlear implant team will be able to advise you on funding options.

## Summary

Cochlear implants, which once provided only sound awareness, now make it possible for many children with limited residual hearing to hear and understand speech and other sounds. Still, as with hearing aids, it takes time and support. For some children progress will be seen more quickly than for others. Particularly for those who have challenges in addition to hearing loss the prognosis may be less certain. For all children adjustments will be needed and it will take time to determine the best map. Be patient: an experienced audiologist, working with other professionals, will offer support and guidance. But it will take dedication and perseverance on your part to seek information, to nurture your child's development of hearing for communication, to maintain the hardware, and to advocate for educational services. If these things can be successfully accomplished, you and your child will be rewarded with access to a world of sound unavailable by any other means.

# 6

# THE CARE AND USE OF HEARING AIDS AND COCHLEAR IMPLANTS

For most hard-of-hearing children, hearing can serve as the primary channel for acquiring speech and language, but only if the proper technology is appropriately fitted and consistently maintained. The amount of benefit from hearing aid use is determined by a variety of factors including the type of hearing loss, amount of hearing loss, and the clarity of amplified sound. The amount of time the equipment is used and the consistency of use are also important variables. Family members, teachers, and caretakers play an important role when it comes to keeping things working properly. Needless to say, the best hearing aids are of little value if the batteries are dead, the earmold is clogged, or the child refuses to wear them.

## Batteries

There's nothing more basic to proper hearing aid use than batteries. Yet discharged or improperly inserted batteries are still a major cause of malfunction. Your audiologist will provide a first set of batteries and a battery tester (Figure 6–1) along with an orientation on how to test and insert the batteries (Figure 6–2). Unlike the batteries in your wristwatch, hearing aid batteries need to be changed frequently. How often depends on the degree of your child's hearing

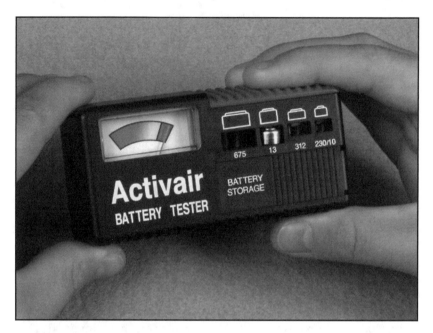

**Figure 6–1.** A battery tester designed for hearing aid batteries.

loss and how the hearing aids are used. You're likely to go through batteries more frequently in cold weather and noisy environments and if your child uses an FM system.

When Elizabeth first began wearing hearing aids, I changed the batteries every 13 days. By the time she was in first grade and using an FM every day, I had to change the batteries once a week. But when she got a new FM at the end of second grade, I suddenly had to change the batteries every 4 days. I couldn't figure out the problem. Neither could the audiologist, so the aids, which were 4 years old, were sent in for reconditioning.

By then it was summer, and because Elizabeth wasn't using the FM, I could go a week or more without changing batteries. But once school began again, so did the annoyingly frequent changes. I met people in the audiology clinic whose children had far greater hearing losses than Elizabeth, and their batteries lasted over a week. What was wrong with ours? After a thorough question-and-answer session with the audiologist, I learned something: the new FM boots sucked power from the hearing aid batteries even when the FM

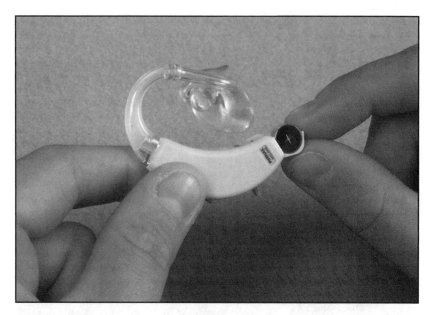

**Figure 6–2.** The hearing aid battery must be properly inserted and the battery door should be tamper resistant.

wasn't being used. After that I began taking the boots off after school. Soon we were back to having batteries last a week.

Batteries are the lifeline for hearing aids. They're also just the right size and shape to be chewed or swallowed. Hearing aids designed for young children have tamper-proof battery doors. It's important to make sure they are properly closed and that batteries not in use are properly stored.

For some children, however, tamper-proof doors aren't protection enough. Long before his 1st birthday, Collin figured out how to pull off his hearing aids and discovered the joy of sucking on them. His saliva short-circuited the on-off switch and leaked into the battery compartment, causing corrosion. It wasn't unusual for the family to go through two sets of batteries a day. His parents cleaned the battery door with a Q-tip dipped in alcohol in an effort to dry the unit, but the damage had been done: the hearing aid had to be sent away for repairs. After that, Collin's audiologist recommended Superseal, a stretchy latex cover that fits over the hearing aid to protect it from moisture.

## Listening Checks

First thing in the morning and as many times as possible through-out the day it's important to attach the hearing aids to a *stethoset* (Figure 6-3) and listen carefully as you repeat various sounds and

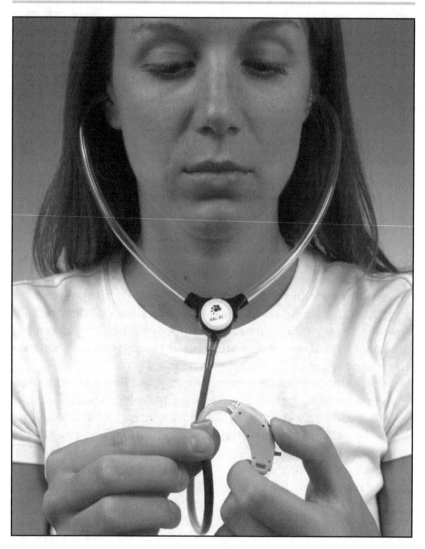

**Figure 6-3.** A stethoset used to perform a listening check on a BTE hearing aid.

phrases. Although it seems a little strange at first to be talking to yourself, with practice you'll become proficient at noticing when things go wrong. A hearing aid with no output is not difficult to detect, but it's also important to notice a loss of clarity or loose connections that cause intermittent output.

## Volume Control

While your child is young you'll need to make sure the volume control stays at the proper setting. Snap-on volume control covers are available and highly recommended to ensure that the hearing aid is not delivering too much or too little amplification.

## Earmolds

To understand the earmold's purpose and pitfalls, it's important to understand how it is intended to work. A channel within the earmold, known as the *sound bore*, contains a short length of plastic tubing. Together, the tubing and earmold carry amplified sounds from the hearing aid to the ear canal.

It all sounds pretty straightforward, but several things can and, at some point, will go wrong. The most common problem is acoustic feedback, the annoying whistling sound familiar to parents, hearing aid users, and anyone who has ever attended a school assembly where a PA system is in use. In the last case, the whistling occurs because the microphone is too close to the speaker, creating a squeal so loud it can be heard in the next county. The cause is overamplification of incoming sound: when the microphone gets too close to the receiver it causes an amplification loop that overloads the amplifier. The only solution, in the case of the PA system, is to lower the volume (which defeats the purpose of the device) or to move the microphone further from the speaker (the appropriate solution).

In some ways a hearing aid is like a miniature PA system. Because the volume level cannot be turned down without defeating its purpose and since the ear is pretty much unmovable, hearing aids use another method to prevent acoustic feedback: the earmold.

The earmold creates a sound barrier between the microphone and receiver. All is well as long as the earmold fits snugly into the external ear and ear canal. But an earmold that is too small or improperly inserted will create a "leak," resulting in acoustic feedback. Feedback can also occur if earwax has accumulated, which will create an obstruction that prevents the amplified sound from passing through the ear canal.

Regardless of the cause, you'll need to take care of the problem. If the mold is loose or not fitting properly, the earmold will likely have to be remade. If the problem is impacted earwax, your child may have to visit the pediatrician, although some audiologists will remove earwax.

Keeping the earmolds clean and properly functioning requires careful inspection and cleaning. Your audiologist may provide you with a small wire loop to help with wax removal (Figure 6-4). If your child's ear is like Elizabeth's and secretes enough wax to discolor a new earmold in 2 weeks, you will need to use it frequently. You can also use a mild detergent, such as dishwashing soap, and a

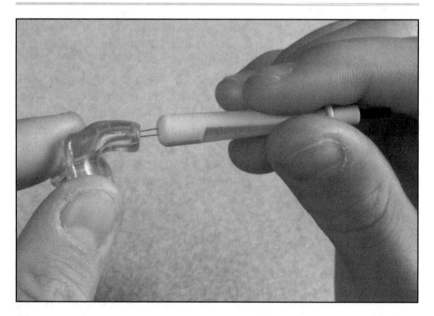

**Figure 6–4.** A small "wax loop" is used to remove debris from the earmold.

damp—not wet—cloth. However, the tubing must first be separated from the hearing aid. With most earmolds the tubing is glued into the sound bore. But where it attaches to the tone hook it is pushed into place (Figure 6-5). After the earmold has been removed and washed, it should be dried before reusing. Blowing through the tubing or using a small squeeze ball designed for this purpose (Figure 6-6) will clear water or other debris trapped in the sound bore. When reattaching the earmold to the hearing aid it's important to make sure you have it pushed securely in place and properly oriented.

## Problems You May Encounter

You may be the most careful and conscientious person in the universe, but when your child spends her waking hours wearing small, fragile, expensive, and highly sophisticated electronic devices, problems will arise. The best advice I can offer is this: expect the

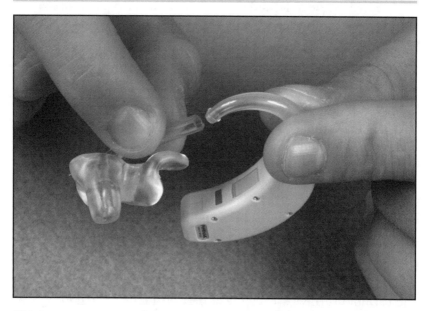

**Figure 6–5.** Attaching the earmold tubing to the hearing aid (the tubing is glued at the other end where it enters the earmold).

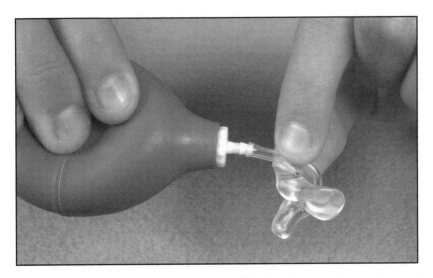

**Figure 6–6.** A squeeze ball is used after cleaning to clear water and debris from the earmold tubing and sound bore.

unexpected; be flexible; and if possible, have backup aids or loaner instruments. Insurance is well worth considering. It also helps to have a sense of humor.

## Acoustic Feedback

The only good thing about acoustic feedback is that we know it's happening. Correcting the problem is not always as easy. Most feedback problems are due to improper insertion; however, young children quickly outgrow their earmolds, resulting in a loose fitting. If the mold is properly inserted and snug with no block or leaks in the earmold tubing, consult your audiologist.

## Earmold Remakes

The earmold is the least technical part of the hearing aid but it is often the weakest link. If your child's ears are full of wax, even the most expensive and sophisticated hearing aids won't help. Likewise, the most optimal hearing aid is useless if the earmold doesn't fit properly. Either the hearing aids will fall out (and risk being lost or trampled upon) or they will whistle continuously.

Babies often outgrow their earmolds within a few weeks. The replacement cycle usually slows down, but during the early years you may feel as if you're spending more time at the audiologist than at the playground. Tell-tale signs that it's time for a new earmold are when they come out or go in too easily, when you can see gaps around the edge of the earmold, when acoustic feedback becomes a regular part of your day, or when the earmold falls out simply because your child has tipped her head to one side or another or rubbed the side of her head against something. When high-power aids are required, however, some feedback is inevitable when hats, hands, or anything else is close to the hearing aid.

Arthur and Tracy's son, Collin, got his first pair of hearing aids when he was 2 months old. The family lives in North Carolina and their audiologist is more than an hour from their home. By the time Collin was 11 months old he was on his sixth set of earmolds and his parents had put a lot of miles on their car.

"The audiologist explained to us that it would happen quickly, because children grow so fast," Arthur says.

On the positive side, Arthur and Tracy have an alternative to photography for chronicling Collin's growth. "We have all the earmolds from the first ones all the way up," Arthur says. "It's amazing to look at the size of them!"

## Impacted Wax (Cerumen)

Recall from Chapter 1 that it's normal to have some earwax on the walls of the ear canal. Obstruction from impacted cerumen is often a problem for hearing aid users because the earmold tends to push the wax back in. Make sure you have your child's ear canals inspected any time there is a medical or audiology appointment. When a significant wax buildup *does* occur it should be removed by an experienced clinician, usually a physician or nurse (some audiologists provide "cerumen management" but most do not). It's best to avoid over-the-counter earwax removal products for children.

## Comments and Advice of Strangers (and Friends!)

No matter how well intentioned, the comments of people on the street, in checkout lines, and in other public places are, at times, unwelcome. Collin was diagnosed shortly after birth with a moderate bilateral sensorineural loss. His sister, Hannah, who is almost 3 years older, took it upon herself to inform the general public. Noticing the stares from an elderly woman with a small child at the grocery store one day, she said, "This is my baby brother, Collin, and he has hearing aids. Your baby doesn't have hearing aids," to which the woman replied, "Thank God." Says Tracy, "I don't think Hannah picked up on it, but it hurt my feelings. I said to Hannah, 'Let's just move on down the aisle. Let's just leave these guys alone.'"

## What Goes in Comes Out

Every parent knows that children love to remove shoes, hats, and other things. The earmold is an easy target because of its convenient location. Fortunately, two factors work in our favor. First of all, most children, once accustomed to their hearing aids, prefer to wear them; in fact, some object strongly when they're taken out. Second, audiologists and suppliers of hearing aid accessories have come up with ingenious ways to retain the devices. Your audiologist can provide Huggie Aids to hold the hearing aids in place and clip-on retention devices to prevent them from getting lost if they do fall out of the ear.

Elizabeth got her first hearing aids on a Friday. The audiologist warned us that there would be an adjustment period. "It will probably take her the weekend to get used to them," she said. "Don't be surprised if she tries to take them out, but remind her, that's your job."

At 3, Elizabeth was too young to be responsible for removing her aids—not that that stopped her. On Friday, she pulled them out repeatedly. To be fair, one episode, during which she yanked them out and fled from the room screaming and crying, occurred immediately after I turned on the vacuum cleaner when she was standing next to it. Important Lesson #1: Do not turn on the vacuum cleaner or any other loud appliance near your newly-aided child. By Saturday she was down to pulling them out a handful of times. By

Sunday, she wanted them in all the time and even protested when we took them out at night.

Not all children will react the same way. Babies especially are notorious for yanking out their hearing aids. But older children, too, will sometimes refuse to wear them, even after months or years of compliance. When that happens, your goal should be to determine the problem. Resist the urge to remind your child that the aids help and she must wear them. If she has been willingly wearing them until this point, she undoubtedly knows they help.

"Fighting is not a good solution," says Brad Ingrao, an audiologist and editor of EDEN, the Electronic Deaf Education Network (info@bradingrao.com). "It sets up a power struggle that you're bound to lose."

Quite often, the reluctance stems from a physical problem. If the output is set too high, the aids will be too loud, which will be uncomfortable. If the output is too low, your child won't hear clearly, which can make the aids seem pointless. In either case, the audiologist needs to be informed of your concerns so settings can be checked.

If your child sweats excessively, the earmolds may be causing discomfort. A cut, sore, or rash can make it painful to wear an earmold. A mild external ear infection or fungus can make the earmold feel itchy. Again, you should consult your audiologist about these problems. In the latter instance, your child may have to leave the aid or aids out until the ear is healed, as having something rubbing against a sore will only prolong the problem.

Kim, who is 42 and has worn hearing aids for her profound sensorineural loss since she was nearly 4, says she always found her earmolds uncomfortable. When she sweated—and as she is an active person, that happens often—the earmolds felt as if they were clogging her ears. When she smiled, which was also often, the aids whistled.

Her problems were solved, she says, when an audiologist concluded that when she smiled, ate, or chewed gum, her jaw joints might be altering the shape of her ear canals where the ends of the molds rested. The audiologist recommended that she use something called Comply Canal Tips, which are made of a soft, foamlike material and act as a cushion to improve comfort and seal. They also absorb moisture, so sweat is less of a problem. Comply Canal Tips should be available at your audiology clinic.

## Moisture Problems

Some children, especially toddlers, enjoy dropping their hearing aids into the toilet, the bathtub, or whatever other body of water is nearby. A few parents have told me about dropping hearing aids into water by accident, usually because one person is handing them to another just before getting into a pool or the tub.

As a toddler, Toby dropped his "with great ceremony" into his milk. Recalls his mother, Vicki, "When I took it in for repair, the receptionist said, 'You really should control him better and not let him do that!' Relations between us were tense for a number of years after that, but in the end we became quite good friends."

Important Lesson #2: Keep hearing aids as far from bodies of water as possible. Sweat can also damage hearing aids. If your child plays sports or sweats a lot in general, you may want to consider purchasing Super-Seals, which should be available at your audiology clinic.

You can dry your hearing aids with a towel, but to make sure all the water is gone you'll need a dehumidifier. One such device, known as a Dri-Aid Kit, is a small container with a *decoset* to absorb the moisture (Figure 6-7). A more expensive option is a Dri and Store unit. Your audiology clinic will have these. In humid environments they are routinely recommended. In a pinch you can also make your own by filling a container with rice and placing the aids inside at night or when they need to be dried out.

## Lost Hearing Aids

Despite the best efforts, hearing aids are sometimes lost. You may be lucky and find them, though it might take time and effort.

Ian lost an aid while helping to cut down a Christmas tree. A branch grabbed it and as he turned, the aid flew off. The family wandered through the snow, hunting in vain for the hearing aid. Eventually they gave up.

"When we got home, Ian and my husband took off the net wrapping and stood the tree up," recalls Ian's mom, Jill. "As they shook the branches to get the tree to fill out, the hearing aid fell out of the tree."

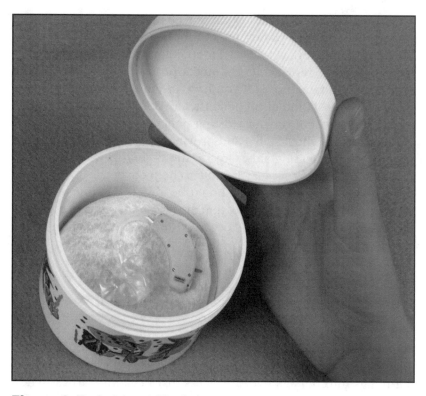

**Figure 6–7.** A dehumidifier helps remove moisture from the hearing aid and earmold.

One mother told me that her son hid one of his aids inside dry-wall. "What fun we had ripping the wall apart to get the aid," she recalls, with more than a bit of irony. Another child hooked his to the springs underneath the front passenger seat in the family car. Yet another hung his on his bike wheels. When his mother went to look for them on the bike, they were gone. "He shrugged and said, 'Must have fallen off,' and was about to go off and play some more," his mother recalls. "I calmly replied, 'You are going *nowhere* until *we find those hearing aids!*'" She enlisted the help of her older son and his friend, who immediately found an aid on the front lawn. They spent 45 minutes searching for the second one, which turned up in the neighbor's front yard—under the sprinkler.

Not every story about lost or banged-up hearing aids will have a happy ending, and paying for the replacements can take a bite out of any family budget. Ask your audiologist about special insurance policies or replacement benefits provided by some hearing instrument manufacturers. If you have insurance on your home or apartment you should also check the cost of adding a hearing aid replacement benefit to your existing policy.

Fortunately, most states and provinces have programs to help parents pay for hearing aids. Organizations such as the Lions Club also have programs that may be able to help cover the cost of your hearing aids. Your audiologist should be able to provide you with information. The Resources section also contains a list of agencies and organizations that can help you with more information about how to pay for hearing aids.

## More Adventures in Amplification

Before Elizabeth got hearing aids, I used to get really upset about things like lost pacifiers and missing mittens. The hearing aids helped put things into perspective, a process that began in earnest when Elizabeth's first aids were 4 months old. I was getting her ready for bed when I discovered she was wearing only one. My stomach lurched, my heart began to pound, and I felt weak and ill. The only place the aid could have been was at the playground, and the playground was a vast, sand-covered expanse which, at 9:30 p.m., even up here above the 53rd parallel in mid-July, wasn't going to be well lit. I left Dave with the kids and fled to the playground where I scoured the sand until I forced myself to admit I was wasting my time.

Then I remembered that Elizabeth had been nodding off to sleep in the car earlier that day. I decided, just for the heck of it, to look around the back seat. Sure enough, there was the hearing aid.

I learned an important lesson that night: if a hearing aid falls out just because your child's head has rubbed up against a car seat, chances are the earmold no longer fits properly. Soon after that incident, we went to the audiologist, who ordered new earmolds for our rapidly growing daughter.

Our next disaster occurred two summers later, when Elizabeth and Noah went swimming at a friend's pool. Dave, who was watching the kids with the friend's dad, left the hearing aids on a bench in the yard. While the kids were in the pool and the dads were chatting, the friend's puppy ate one of the hearing aids. By the time Dave discovered what had happened, all that remained was the earmold (which was apparently indigestible), a shred of flesh-colored plastic casing, and bits of unidentifiable masticated electronics. The dog was throwing up, which is what I felt like doing when I returned home and got the news.

I was certain that our insurance rider would cover the cost, but how was I going to explain to the audiologist that we'd been so careless?

"Oh, don't worry," the receptionist told me when I called. "This sort of thing happens all the time."

In fact, when we brought what was left of the hearing aid to the clinic the next day, one of the mothers in the waiting room told me the same thing had happened to her son's aid years earlier. I was so relieved to know I wasn't alone that I pulled the shredded plastic out of my pocket to show her.

"Oh my!" she said, her eyes wide with surprise. "Ours wasn't nearly that bad!"

William wears a hearing aid only in his right ear. His left ear has no residual hearing, so there's no point in aiding that ear. As a toddler, he once yanked off his hearing aid in the grocery store, pulled it apart, and threw it under a shelving unit. His mom, Cindy, had to crawl under the unit to retrieve it.

Another time she took William and his older sister to the beach in their home state of North Carolina for a weekend. Her husband was to meet the family there. The night before he arrived, Cindy realized William's aid was missing.

"There was a guy on the beach with a metal detector," she recalls. "I asked him if he had come across a hearing aid. He hadn't. I walked back and forth from the restaurant to the hotel trying to find it. I was in tears the whole time."

The next day Cindy called the audiologist to report the missing aid and ask for a loaner. "If he had two hearing aids, even if he lost one it'd be all right, but because that is the only one, if it's gone, it's gone," she says.

Cindy has vivid memories of how anxious she felt. "You're short of breath, you feel like you're going to start crying to the man with the metal detector, you're trying to hold it together with these two children standing there, and afterwards you start to think, I need to start signing with this kid. What if? What if? What if? What if? Is that my only mode of communication with him? Is that my only way to reach him, this piece of technology that may or may not be there?"

Cindy's husband arrived that night. He was the one who found the aid, under her overnight bag in the bathroom. "It was another set of eyes, another perspective," she says. "Why, in all of this, I didn't pick it up and look underneath it I don't know."

Another time the aid went missing at a garden center in Seattle, during a visit to Cindy's mother. William had been taking off his hearing aid that day and throwing it around, but it wasn't until they left the center that Cindy realized it was missing.

"We went back but it was already closed," Cindy recalls. "So I climbed the fence. My mother was outside with her two dogs and my two kids. I'm trespassing. I'm breaking the law. I'm going through the garbage. I pictured what would happen if the police came: 'Ma'am, why don't you steal a plant instead of just rifling through the garbage?'

"The next day we found it," Cindy says. "It was one of those 5:00-in-the-morning things—I remembered he'd taken it off on her deck and thrown it through the slats.

"When you do lose it, that's all you can think about, and then you think, Phew, another close call. But really, how many close calls can your heart take?"

Toby was 2 when he got his first pair of hearing aids more than 20 years ago. It was June, and his brother, who is 5 years older, remembers that he and his parents spent much of the summer on their hands and knees, hunting for hearing aids. They got into the habit of looking into Toby's ears almost constantly, remembering where they were when they saw the aids, so that when they looked again and the inevitable had occurred—that is, Toby had pulled them off and tossed them—they'd have a better idea of how far to backtrack.

"We pawed at many a sand pile, grassy park, and all over the house," Vicki says. "The best was when he parked them in the elevator of his Fisher-Price parking garage. Luckily, they squealed, but it took many hours to find them, and I was sure they'd been flushed down the toilet."

When you're in the midst of a hearing aid crisis, it's hard to imagine you'll ever find the memory amusing. For most parents, though, that's exactly what happens: we take the experience and turn it into an anecdote. Even at the moment I learned that a dog had devoured Elizabeth's hearing aid, I kept calm by repeating to myself, "This is going to be a great story someday." A few years later, when an FM boot disappeared seemingly into thin air, and we spent a week unsuccessfully attempting to find it by retracing our steps, I told myself the same thing. Knowing we had replacement insurance certainly helped me to maintain a level head, but my experiences reminded me, yet again, of the power of humor. Both stories are guaranteed to get a laugh, and the lost boot tale has an added element of surprise. The day after I filed the insurance claim, Elizabeth's former kindergarten teacher found the boot in the first grade classroom, under the teacher's desk. As a result, our story had the happiest ending possible for everyone involved: we got to cancel the claim.

## Cochlear Implant Care and Maintenance

Children who use cochlear implants typically started out as hearing aid users, so by the time of implantation most parents are familiar with small electronic devices, batteries, and the challenges of keeping everything in good working order. Some of the issues related to care and maintenance of cochlear implants are similar to those for hearing aids. Batteries are again the lifeline, but unlike most hearing aids, cochlear implants use rechargeable batteries. Earmolds are used only to hold the device in place, so a snug fit is less critical than it is with hearing aids. And since there's no amplification of sounds, feedback is not an issue.

As noted earlier, there are only a few manufacturers of cochlear implants. Each company provides instructions for care, maintenance, and trouble shooting. If your child gets a cochlear implant your audiologist will make sure you have a supply of extra batteries, cables, and other replacement parts. As with hearing aids, moisture is a potential problem so the Dri-Aid Kit is again a big help.

# 7

# ACCEPTING THE INCOMPREHENSIBLE

In one of my early efforts to understand what it would be like to not hear well, I stuck my fingers into my ears and tried to make out what was being said around me. If Elizabeth had been blind, I probably would have walked around with a scarf tied over my eyes. If she'd been unable to walk, I'd have tried getting around in a wheelchair. But hearing loss isn't something you can try on. Even with my ears plugged, I can hear my own voice clearly, and my brain will automatically adjust to the reduced sound levels so I can focus on what I want to hear.

Two things ultimately helped me understand how Elizabeth could hear: an audiotape designed to simulate the aided hearing of a person with hearing loss (see Resources) and Elizabeth's audiogram coupled with an audiogram that showed the pitch and decibel level of speech and other sounds (see Figure 2-1).

The labels assigned to degree of hearing loss—mild, moderate, moderately severe, severe, profound—are just that: labels. Two children can have similar audiograms but hear very differently. To best help your child, you need to know and understand the audiogram (what it does and does not tell you) and the relationship of the audiogram to speech.

It was only after Elizabeth's audiologist charted her audiogram on the sound banana (a banana-shaped diagram that shows where speech sounds fall on the audiogram) that I was able to better understand how her hearing worked—or, more precisely, how it didn't. Most speech sounds fell out of her hearing range. Unless whoever was talking spoke loudly and clearly, many of the speech sounds would be barely audible to her. Given that words are made up of a series of sounds, it was safe to say that until she was aided, she hadn't been able to hear *anything* loudly or clearly. Again, I was left marveling at how she had managed to develop any kind of working vocabulary and comprehensible speech patterns—and feeling grateful for, instead of self-conscious about, my often loud speaking voice.

Hearing aids can and do help children with mild, moderate, and moderately severe losses. They can also benefit some children with severe hearing loss, but even aided, most children with severe loss won't hear as well as aided children with milder losses. Studies have shown that many children with cochlear implants actually hear more clearly than those who use hearing aids, although sounds are less natural. In general, hearing aids provide less benefit to children with the most severe hearing losses; indeed, such children are generally considered the best candidates for cochlear implants. But some children with cochlear implants, especially those implanted later in life after years of not hearing, either because they were not aided or not aided successfully, will still elect to use manual communication and the services of an interpreter, translator, or transliterator.

What hearing technology or interpreters your child needs, what resources will benefit him, and how he will fare are highly individual. What is universal is that as parents of children who are hard of hearing we must make accommodations. The tangible ones such as getting hearing aids or a cochlear implant, choosing a form of communication, getting closed captioning for the television, buying an alarm clock that shakes the bed instead of buzzes, and getting either a TTY phone or a speakerphone are straightforward. If your audiologist can't help you find the services or equipment you need, consult one of the organizations in the Resources section. All are excellent sources of help.

The adjustments we must make to our expectations aren't as simple. Fears are common in the immediate aftermath of a diagnosis. Sometimes, in retrospect, they can seem irrational, unrealistic, or even amusing. "I remember my eyes welling up with tears on the way home from the audiologist," Elyse says. "My first thought was how tough it would be for Julie to get married."

Julie was 4 years old at the time.

"Are kids going to pick on him at school?" Arthur wondered after his son, Collin, was diagnosed with a moderate hearing loss.

Collin was 6 days old.

My worries took a while to crystallize because I was in denial for more than a month after Elizabeth's initial diagnosis. I had convinced myself that the audiologist was wrong. If he was wrong, I could continue with all my hopes and dreams about my daughter, that she'd learn to play a musical instrument, excel at school, have lots of friends, graduate from college, and have a fabulous career in some white collar profession like her parents and grandparents and aunts and uncles.

Dave, meanwhile, convinced himself that her future was bleak, that she might be mildly retarded or, at the very least, a slow learner. There was no evidence that Elizabeth had any brain damage but, Dave pointed out, the inner ear was connected to the brain, and if that was damaged and we didn't know how, there was a chance her brain was damaged as well. I was furious with him: it was bad enough he had to think that way, but did he have to verbalize those thoughts and plant them in my head, too? And what if he was right? What did it say about us, that we were such elitist snobs that we couldn't bear the thought of parenting an academically challenged child?

Initially to ease my fears, and later as part of research for the first edition of this book, I set out to learn all I could about hearing loss and how hard-of-hearing children learn. Much of that information is covered in Chapter 10. Once Elizabeth got aided and began working with a speech-language pathologist and attending preschool, it became apparent that Dave and I could revise our expectations once again, this time upward. But as any parent discovers, even when hearing loss isn't involved, we're constantly revising our expectations: none of us can predict the future, and lives can change in a second.

Those initial fears inevitably give way to more pressing day-to-day concerns as we try to determine which of our children's behaviors stem from the hearing loss and which are personality traits or reactions to particular situations. Finding a balance between coddling our children and acknowledging how their hearing loss affects their lives is an ongoing challenge. Experts who work with and study children with hearing loss have noted that some have a high level of stress, poor self-esteem, and a low threshold for frustration; they tire easily and respond slowly to directions. Admittedly, there are plenty of children with normal hearing who have those same traits. But understanding how hearing loss contributes to them may help you to better respond, if and when they become a factor in your child's life.

## Listening Can Be Work!

Listening takes more effort when you're trying to hear above background noises that include such potential distractions as fans blowing, feet tapping, music playing, or people talking. That's why your hard-of-hearing child may be more tired when he comes home from school or social activities, why he may require down time after participating in activities that involve other people, and why he may be reluctant to bounce from one event to another and need more sleep.

When Elizabeth was in first grade, a lot of her friends stayed at school for lunch, and she wanted to as well. I thought it was silly: after all, we live only three blocks away and I was home all day, ready to make a nice, hot meal she could eat in the comfort of her own home. But for her it was a social event, so I signed her up for one day a week.

At the end of the first month, I asked if I should sign her up for the rest of the year. "No," she told me. "I don't want to go back. It's too noisy."

I wondered what would happen when she began attending junior high, which was too far to come home for lunch, and had six times as many students as her elementary school. I promised myself that if the lunch room was too loud, I'd talk to school officials about making accommodations so she could eat somewhere quiet and have the down time she needed to be able to function at her best.

As it turned out, my junior high lunchroom fears were unfounded: Elizabeth's junior high has no lunchroom. Usually she eats with a small group of friends in the hall near their lockers. It's noisier than our kitchen, but quieter than the gathering area where the other students eat. And it's taught me some more important lessons: if we provide our children with problem-solving skills, they'll use them. Also, what bothers them in early elementary school won't necessarily prove problematic 6 years down the line. As our children grow, everything about them changes, including their tolerance levels.

## Things Take Time

Auditory processing involves several steps that include sound detection, discrimination, retrieval of relevant information from the brain, and comprehension—remembering what's being said, and understanding it. For people with normal hearing, and even hard-of-hearing infants aided shortly after birth, auditory processing often develops automatically. Later-identified individuals, those with more severe hearing losses, or those with disabilities in addition to hearing loss may have to consciously learn the processes of sound awareness, discrimination, recognition, and comprehension. It's only natural that the process is slower than it is with a person who has normal hearing.

Elizabeth's teachers in early elementary school told me they often repeated instructions for her. As she grew older, that didn't seem to happen as frequently, partly because her listening skills had improved and partly because she learned to advocate for herself and could ask if she wasn't sure about something. I asked her recently what she does if she misses part of what a teacher has said. "Either I can figure out what I've missed by what else the teacher says, or I ask someone," she said.

## Communication Can Sometimes Be Frustrating

Hearing loss is a communication disorder, and not being able to communicate can be stressful and frustrating. Compounding the situation is the fact that the majority of children who wear hearing aids may look and act like everyone else. The result is that folks communicating with them assume they're hearing like everyone else.

A variety of factors affect a child's language comprehension ability, including distance from the person speaking, levels of room noise, and complexity of the language being used, according to leading audiology researcher Mark Ross, himself severely hard of hearing. In *Our Forgotten Children: Hard of Hearing Children in the Public Schools*, he writes, "Adults assume that [children] will comprehend a message because they can so evidently hear it. Other children may consider them less than desirable playmates for reasons that neither group really comprehends" (Ross, 2001). The resulting disparities between what society expects and what hard-of-hearing children are capable of, as well as the conflicts between their needs and the way their needs are often ignored by what Ross calls "an insensitive and ignorant environment," can affect the children throughout their school years and beyond.

Paige got her first set of hearing aids in 1965 when she was 3 years old. They seemed to amplify everything, so she still had trouble picking out the main source of speech. Despite her loss—profound in her left ear, severe in her right—she was an A student. Socially, however, she considered herself a failure.

"What I remember is the frustration of never being able to connect with anyone," she says. "Playing games was hopeless. I could never follow the rules, ever. Somebody would stand up and say, 'these are the rules and you have to do this and this.' It was completely lost on me. What would have helped is if someone had backed up a bit and said, 'Hey, we're playing a game. Do you want to play? Here are the rules,' instead of throwing me into it."

It's heartbreaking to see your child excluded. I remember being on the playground late one afternoon, long after the final school bell had rung. Elizabeth was in second grade. Three girls from her class were playing together. They were assertive, popular girls, the ones with whom she'd never quite fit in. They were also the only people on the playground, so she approached them and asked if she could join their game. I stood back and watched as she had a brief conversation with the girls, who then took off and ran away from her. Elizabeth came back to me, her head down, dejected. She told me they'd said she couldn't play. But had they? Or had she misheard? I sent her back again, and watched as the same scenario unfolded. Finally, the third time, I went to the girls and told them Elizabeth wanted to play, and could they please include her. They did.

When your child is too young to advocate for himself, it's important that you remember, and let those communicating with your child know, that speech needs to be delivered at a slower pace, and the child and whoever is speaking need to be face to face; it's all the skills that are pretty much in place when you communicate with someone who is hard of hearing as an adult.

It's especially important to advocate for your child when he starts school. You'll learn more about how to do that in Chapter 9 and Chapter 10. But whenever your child begins a new activity, whether it's school, sports, Girl Scouts or Boy Scouts, youth group, or even attending a birthday party, you should try to meet in advance with the person in charge, to explain your child's hearing loss and what accommodations are needed.

If your child doesn't have other disabilities, chances are you'll be intervening less and less as he gets older. As he develops the confidence and skills to speak for himself, you won't have to navigate playground friendships—and he won't want you to, anyway. There will still be times when you'll have to advocate, but you'll no doubt be operating more behind the scenes—meeting with teachers at the start of each year of middle school or junior high or high school, and with coaches and other leaders as needed.

## Staying Positive

You don't need to have a hearing loss to suffer low self-esteem. But the fact is, if your child has a hearing loss, at some point he may feel bad about himself and about his hearing loss. In order to help him accept that this is something he'll likely have to deal with for the rest of his life, it's critical that you accept it, too.

Paige says she spent much of her childhood and early adult life pretending she didn't have a hearing loss. It wasn't that anyone came out and told her that a disability was bad. But when a doctor incorrectly concluded that Paige's hearing was normal, her mother's delighted reaction made it apparent that normal hearing made people happy, and hearing loss was cause for gloom. "The underlying message was that it was bad," Paige said. "And the way I was treated by kids at school made it even more clear."

Paige's mother's reaction is understandable—it's a rare parent who hasn't sat in the audiologist's office praying the test results are wrong. But because children are especially sensitive to their parents' feelings and reactions, we need to be aware of and moderate how we cope with our child's hearing loss.

"A hearing aid doesn't have to be embarrassing—it's not," says Carren Stika, PhD, a clinical psychologist in San Diego who was diagnosed with a progressive hearing loss when she was 22. Carren has a long track record of working with hearing-impaired children and their parents, in private practice and in conducting psychoeducational evaluations for school districts, the courts, and the House

Ear Institute in Los Angeles. She also teaches a course in pediatric and aural rehabilitation at San Diego State University.

In Carren's experience, the embarrassment is generally more a reflection of the parents, who feel their child is defective. Rather than focus on the hearing aid, she says, it's important to help a child build his self-esteem.

"Hearing loss doesn't have to be a curse," she says. "It doesn't mean you can't have a life or succeed. What it means is a parent has to be able to find out, how can we help this child and how can we not make this into more than it has to be? How do we see our child beyond the hearing loss, that life and life's tasks and successes are multiple?

"A mild hearing loss or a moderate hearing loss or a severe hearing loss does not have to be a major disability as long as it's handled properly. It runs in close partnership with how those who are serving the child are responding to the hearing loss."

That doesn't mean you have to love the hearing aid or cochlear implant. In fact, you're likely to have a love-hate relationship with all of your child's equipment, which, when it's working properly, can do wonders and when it's not can be seriously disruptive. What it does mean is that each of us has to find the balance between acknowledging our children's very real frustration when they come to us (as they will) with some variation of "Why do I have to wear hearing aids? Nobody else does," and keeping them from wallowing in self-pity.

When 42-year-old Kim was growing up, she often removed her hearing aids. It was bad enough that she was the only kid in school who wore them, but they whistled constantly, which drew even more unwanted attention. The self-consciousness evaporated only when she began attending a residential school for the deaf, where nearly everyone wore hearing aids.

Putting your child in an environment where everyone is just like her—removing her from the mainstream—is a solution, but it's not going to work for everyone. And there are other ways to help your child realize he's not unique (or strange, weird, different, or whatever adjective he chooses to describe himself on a particular day).

One of the most critical factors is to make sure, from an early age, that your child has role models who wear hearing aids, says Florida audiologist Brad Ingrao. "They should know several adults who demonstrate that wearing hearing aids improves their ability to communicate and thereby to show the world their best. If they can look to these role models, they may be less likely to let the fact that other kids don't wear hearing aids really bother them."

Brad, who has a son who is deaf and uses American Sign Language (ASL), also stresses the importance of helping children understand their hearing loss and the power that their aids gives them to control their environment.

Toby, 28, who has worn hearing aids since he was 2 years old, says the best advice for parents is "have faith, be supportive, and don't panic—it's not the end of the world."

A graduate of a technical college in Toronto, Toby is a cameraman at a television station in the city. "I look at myself and I've done quite well for my age. I have friends who aren't doing much of anything—they're not deaf or anything, they just don't know what they want to do."

Jenny, who received a cochlear implant when she was 16 and now works as a quality assurance analyst, says one of the best things her parents did for her and her sister, who is also deaf, was to support them and make sure their needs were met without putting unnecessary emphasis on their hearing losses.

"They came along with me to speech therapies, helped me to correct my speech, supported me when I wanted the cochlear implant and, basically, made me feel very special," she says. "I believe it is extremely important that parents of hearing-impaired children treat their child just like any normal hearing child, and not highlight their disability. It does wonders for their self-esteem. I know, being hard of hearing is not something to be ashamed of, or something to hide, but when you are 10 years old, you tend to want to fit in with your peers at school and, therefore, it's important to be one of them."

Parents who also have normal-hearing children have another challenge: to ensure that those children aren't shunted to the side because of the special needs of the hard-of-hearing child.

Terri, a mom in Virginia, found herself with little choice but to devote nearly all her time and attention to her hard-of-hearing baby, Caleb, who spent the first month of his life in the neonatal intensive care unit of a university hospital in the neighboring state of North Carolina.

Terri and her husband, Wayne, had two older daughters, 11-year-old Rachel and 8-year-old Sarah. Caleb had severe disabilities and his medical needs took nearly all of Terri's time. Her mother and her friends helped out a lot, but they couldn't make up for her absence in her daughters' lives.

The girls "would tell me they missed me or they needed me to 'love on them'—they'd come up to me and say, 'I need some loving, Mom,'" Terri recalls. "Sarah had to grow up so fast, and Rachel did, too. Wayne was working 60 to 70 hours a week and our life was in a whirlwind. They adjusted. They had to. There was no balance in our family during that first year—it was basically just a matter of trying to survive it all."

By the time he was 3 months old, Caleb was fitted with hearing aids and glasses. He traveled with an oxygen tank, and he attracted a lot of attention. The girls' reactions to him were as profound as they were different. Sarah, the youngest, welcomed the attention and mothered Caleb. Rachel, the oldest, was scared of this baby who projectile-vomited without warning. When they went out in public, she felt embarrassed.

"At that age, the one thing you don't want is attention all the time," Terri says. "Every time we went somewhere, we were stared at and people would just come up and want to know about him. People would walk by and touch him, blessing him."

Terri told Rachel to look her best "because we knew people would be looking at us—not many people had seen a baby that little with hearing aids, glasses, and oxygen."

"Her life changed a lot," Terri recalls. "I couldn't be there like I was before. It was a very stressful time at our house. She managed to remain a straight-A student in all advanced classes. I don't know how. She missed the life we had before Caleb was born. It was so much easier, and we didn't even know it."

Psychotherapist Jeanne Safer, author of *The Normal One: Life with a Difficult or Damaged Sibling* (2003), advises parents to allow nondisabled children to express negative feelings about a sibling with disabilities, even if it upsets the parents. "Don't require them always to 'understand'—they're children," she says.

She strongly recommends setting aside time for nondisabled siblings and letting them be the center of attention regularly. Praise their achievements so they realize they, too, are important.

"Let them have their own friends, their own activities, and their own moments to shine."

Jeanne also counsels that normal-hearing siblings shouldn't be expected to share their parents' feelings or level of involvement with a sibling who has disabilities. "Being a sibling is different from being a parent."

Ultimately, of course, parents will decide what works best for their families. California parents Alicia and Bill already had two toddlers at home when they learned that their baby, Sylvia, was deaf. After researching communication options, they decided Sylvia should receive a cochlear implant and learn oral skills.

"We have two other children and we had to take them into account," Alicia says. "We felt really, really strongly that we didn't want them to be responsible to translate for her. We felt that if we went for sign language, they'd have to constantly be translating for her, and we didn't want to put that on them—that's not fair to them."

Sylvia received a cochlear implant in her left ear when she was 12½ months old. By the time she was 2 she had no trouble speaking for herself, more proof to her parents that they'd made the right decision. When Sylvia was 3½, she received an implant in her right ear. She's now 7 years old, mainstreamed, and at the top of her class in school.

Caleb, who just turned 8, is also a straight-A student. It's a trait he shares with his oldest sister, who has come to appreciate him, not just for his work in school, but for his charm, his outgoing personality, and his artistic talent. Before Rachel went off to college, she would bring school friends home and Caleb was always the first person her friends visited with.

"Everybody wanted to see and talk to Caleb because he was so interesting and into so many different things," Terri says, and it's impossible not to hear the pride and happiness in her voice. "The kids couldn't believe his artwork. Everyone in our home and their friends and our friends have grown to love him. It makes people really happy because they see what he can do. It's made Rachel not afraid, not embarrassed, but very proud of who he has become, of his accomplishments."

In 2007, Rachel graduated second in her high school class. She earned so many scholarships that her first year of college was paid for. Many of her application essays were about life with Caleb.

"All the things we went through, all the hardships, just dealing with having someone in our family with a disability, the way it changed us, has come back and rewarded us over and over and it's made us stronger and more prepared for life," Terri says. "The big thing that we understand and we'll continue to understand is that it's not all about perfect, it's about being happy and even though things are not perfect and fit perfectly into a mold, it's taking what you have and being happy with your life. That's what we've accomplished as a family."

## Adjustment: A Lifelong Process

There is no one path to acceptance and adjustment, and neither is it a one-shot deal. Just when you think you've got everything under control, a piece of equipment will fail, something will get lost or broken, or a teacher, coach, or classmate will make an ignorant comment. Every time your child enters a new class or a new school, joins a team, goes to camp, or begins a new activity you'll need to re-explain his hearing loss and what accommodations are necessary. You may feel as if you're repeating yourself, but the information is new to the people you're addressing, and they need to hear it as much as the last several thousand people for whom you've covered the territory. If your child has a progressive or fluctuating hearing loss, you'll have to adjust each time the audiogram changes.

Jill, whose son, Ian, was diagnosed at age 7 with a progressive bilateral conductive hearing loss, had accepted the condition and incorporated the new reality of hearing aids, doctor's visits, and FM into the family routine. Then, when he was 12, Ian's doctors began to suspect he also had cochlear damage that would eventually leave him with no hearing. The news threw Jill into a tailspin.

The reality that the loss was gradual meant that the family would have time to adapt, but at the same time, Jill feared the news would devastate her son. "I know that for parents whose kids have been born deaf or who have lost hearing at a much younger age, this may sound harsh, but completely losing his hearing and knowing it is a certainty is going to be very hard on this kid, as well as us as parents," she said not long after the diagnosis.

She was only half right. When Ian learned his progressive sensorineural loss made him a candidate for a cochlear implant, he told his mother that was cool.

"He thinks it will be great to have 'bionic ears,'" Jill says. "Me? I cried when I heard the news. He took it completely in stride."

As it turned out, Ian wasn't a candidate for an implant: tests showed that his cochlea was healthy. His loss, as doctors had correctly diagnosed when he was 7, is almost entirely conductive, and it's caused by otosclerosis. The disease is slowly immobilizing the bones in his middle ear.

When Ian was a child, his parents had considered an operation called a stapedectomy, where his stapes bone would be replaced with a prosthetic. Because of his age, the procedure was considered too risky. Doctors recommended waiting until after puberty, when his physiology had matured and the risks would be diminished.

The spring that Ian turned 16, he expressed an interest in learning more about the surgery. Puberty for boys continues long past 16, but Ian's parents brought him to a surgeon anyway. She had performed more than 300 stapedectomies and she was very clear to Ian about the risks: he could lose all the hearing in that ear. Doctors don't always know why, but in about one out of 100 people who have the surgery, the cochlea is damaged.

"Essentially it dies," Jill says. "One percent doesn't sound like very bad odds, but it's a very bad outcome."

The surgeon told Ian she felt he didn't need to take the risk. "He's a successful hearing aid user, his attitude about his hearing loss is a healthy one, and he has no problem using an FM and other assistive devices," Jill says. "For kids who refuse to use their devices, or who feel ostracized, the risks may be worthwhile. But for Ian, she point-blank told him it was rather amazing how well-adjusted he was to his situation."

Ian asked the surgeon how many of her more than 300 patients had lost their hearing. "None," she said.

And then, as if to prove just how well-adjusted he was, Ian said, "After you get three people who lose their hearing, I'll come to see you, but right now your odds are not in my favor."

The surgeon told Ian to take 2 weeks to make a decision, but he made up his mind before he got home from her office. He didn't want the operation.

"It wasn't because he's afraid of becoming more deaf," Jill says. "He fully expects to become more deaf as his loss progresses. He decided not to do it because he knows how to be *his* kind of deaf. He knows how to function successfully in school—how to be a good student. He is going to college next year, and if he suddenly became completely deaf in one ear, he'd have to learn very quickly to become *that* kind of deaf. As it stands now, his loss will progress, and he'll adjust as it happens."

Carolyn's son, Darrell, now in his early 20s, was diagnosed at a year with a profound hearing loss. He now has a cochlear implant. Carolyn believes in perseverance. "Never give up!" she says. "Make your house and yard the fun place to go so lots of children will want to come and play. Educate the people around your child. Aim high. Never believe what the so-called 'professionals' think your child can or cannot achieve. We were told 'Your son probably will never hear,' even after 10 years of wearing hearing aids, and 'He will graduate with the equivalent of a grade six education.' Our son graduated 4 months after his peers—with a high school education."

"Dare to ask questions if you don't understand something," says Janet, whose son, Kevin, was left profoundly deaf after a bout with meningitis when he was a year old. He now has a cochlear implant. "At the end, the parents know the child better than any other person in the world. This doesn't mean not to be open to advice—the professionals always know a lot, but they don't always know better. We are the parents, and we are the ones making the decisions and taking the consequences for those decisions."

"Expect a roller coaster ride of emotions as your child grows," another mother told me. "You'll go from one extreme to the other and back again. It's okay, but just keep going. Keep learning. Keep involved—and more importantly than all that, let your child be a child first. Let them ride bikes, take dance lessons or gymnastics, swim and join sports and anything else they have an interest in."

Karen, whose daughter, Christina, began wearing hearing aids for her severe bilateral loss at 6 months and received a cochlear implant at age 7, says the best advice she can give is that which was passed along to her when Christina was diagnosed: "Give yourself permission to grieve, for as long as you need, whenever you need it. Then, put your heart aside and get down to the business of making the most out of this situation. You will see after some time that you actually say out loud, 'It's okay. Hearing loss is not the end of the world.'"

### Connecting With Other Parents

*When the parents of children with hearing loss are asked about their most important resources for information and emotional support, they often report "other parents." Opportunities to connect with other families range from support groups sponsored by a university or speech and hearing center, to groups organized by the parents themselves.*

*The Internet has opened new doors for parent-to-parent communication, but most families still prefer direct contact. Some are able to combine the two by bringing kids and families together for occasional gatherings and then using email to communicate. Others prefer to connect with only one or two families as they work through the process of learning and acceptance. Ask your audiologist and other service providers for recommendations on how you can meet other parents. Even if there are no formal support groups in your area, many audiologists maintain a list of parents who have agreed to serve as a resource to other parents. Also, you will be able to connect with parents through some of the organizations and web sites listed in the Resources section.*

# 8

# HEARING LOSS AS A PART OF DAILY LIFE

In the initial days and weeks after a diagnosis, it's hard for many of us to believe our lives will get back to whatever sort of normal they were before. It seems unrealistic to imagine that hearing loss will someday cease to become the center of our universe, that it can and will become part of our routine, like brushing our teeth, grocery shopping, or doing the laundry.

Yet it will—it has to, because our children are more than "walking hearing aids," a phrase coined by Jenny, the college student quoted in Chapter 7. When you think about it, it's ironic that the diagnosis seems so devastating: our initial reaction tends to be that everything about our children has changed for the worse when, in fact, the news should be cause for optimism. Our children have been hearing poorly, in some cases for years, and now they'll be able to hear and communicate that much better.

Admittedly, it's a lot easier for me to look at things that way now. When Elizabeth was diagnosed, what was particularly overwhelming was the realization that Dave and I had to revise our expectations for her, but because we had no experience with childhood hearing loss and therefore no idea what we were up against, we had no clue where to begin. We were fortunate in that we were referred almost immediately to the local rehabilitation hospital and provided with a "team"—an audiologist, a pediatric otolaryngologist, a speech-language pathologist, and a social worker who helped us navigate through the paperwork from the different agencies that offered services for disabled children and their families. The social worker also referred us to local, national, and international support groups and agencies. Those groups and others are listed in the Resources section.

Not everyone will have a support team assembled for them. However, even if you have to do it on your own, it's critical that you find the people to help you and your child to understand and attend to the hearing loss and the role it will play in your lives. If your audiologist can't refer you to proper pediatric specialists and support groups, refer to the Resources section, which has a list of agencies and organizations designed to put parents in touch with the appropriate personnel or groups.

When it comes to emotional support, other parents who have been through what you're experiencing are your best resource. One of the most consistent pieces of advice I received from parents and professionals while researching this book was to get to know other parents of hard-of-hearing children, and to make sure your child gets to know other children and adults with hearing aids or cochlear implants. If you don't have the time or inclination to join a support group, or if none exists in your area, consider getting to know people through one of the Internet listservs, chat rooms, or bulletin boards offered by some of the groups in the Resources section.

I tend to be outgoing, and so after I had finally accepted that Elizabeth's hearing loss was real and permanent, I began talking to just about everyone I saw with hearing aids. I struck up conversations with parents in the audiology clinic, senior citizens standing in line buying batteries at Radio Shack, and a mother at Disneyland whose two young children were wearing green and orange hearing aids (a revelation, as I'd assumed beige was the only available color).

From these casual conversations, I learned all sorts of things, among them that our prolonged odyssey to figure out what was wrong with Elizabeth's hearing wasn't unusual, that kids with mild-to-moderate hearing losses didn't necessarily go through batteries at the same rate, and that even earmolds come in a variety of colors. Almost invariably, people were pleasant, helpful, interested, and sometimes downright chatty. Perhaps they were polite by nature, or maybe I reminded them of a time when they, too, were struggling with this new reality, and someone had also helped them.

Other parents can offer so much, from support and comfort to practical suggestions. "One of the most useful things we did shortly after our daughter's diagnosis was to have a family with a daughter who was deaf over for dinner," said Matthew and Pamela, whose daughter, Sophia, received a cochlear implant before she turned 2. "We asked them a hundred questions or more and learned so much! Their daughter was amazing—she's also a cochlear implant user— and was making exceptional progress." After that dinner, Matthew and Pamela began bringing Sophia to a monthly playgroup for children with hearing loss.

I looked into joining a support group, but when Elizabeth was enrolled in preschool for hard-of-hearing children I realized I already had one: the parents of her classmates. The teachers encouraged us to attend so we could see what our children were learning and reinforce their lessons at home. Most of the parents worked full-time. Because my schedule was flexible I showed up regularly. So did Gwen, the grandmother of Nikki, the little girl whose speech had so impressed Rachel, Elizabeth's speech-language pathologist. Nikki was the only other girl in the class, and she and Elizabeth liked each other a lot. They had similar interests: music, art, and animals, and they played easily together. Neither seemed impatient about repeating something if the other couldn't hear, which doesn't always happen with Elizabeth's hearing friends.

Gwen and I also developed a good friendship. During school we would occasionally steal off to an observation room to trade stories, and when we got the girls together outside of school, the play dates were as rewarding for us as they were for the children.

Every few months, the parent liaison at the school organized a meeting where all the parents could get together, and it was there that I learned even more: that some kids were allergic to earmolds, that batteries didn't work as efficiently in cold weather, that other people's equipment broke down at least as often as ours did. From the parent liaison, the mother of a teenage son who was deaf, we learned that things wouldn't necessarily get easier as the years went on, but they would be, at the very least, different, and that the skills we were learning now would prepare us for what was to come.

How we come to accept and adjust to our child's hearing loss depends on so many factors: the age of our child at the time of the diagnosis, our family situation, our general outlook on life, where we live, what supports are available to us, whether we've had experience with other disabilities. One reason support groups, listservs, and chat rooms are so useful is that it's always helpful to hear about other people's experiences.

## Becky: Hearing Loss Wasn't Such a Big Deal

"I think the thing that makes me different from everybody else is that I have an older child with a disability," says my neighbor, Kathy, whose youngest daughter, Becky, is a year younger than Elizabeth and was diagnosed at age 3 with a mild-to-moderate high-frequency hearing loss.

Kathy has five other daughters. Her second oldest, Elfi, who is 12 years older than Becky, was born with spina bifida and had the first of more than a dozen operations when she was 1 day old.

"Becky's disability wasn't life threatening—Elfi's was," Kathy says. "We weren't sure she was going to come through right away —she had to have her back closed. There's an extreme loss of control when your child is having so many surgeries. It's a much more severe thing to cope with, I thought, than simply having to put in some hearing aids right away."

Although Kathy's instinct is to minimize the hearing loss, she has no intention of ignoring it. "If I'd known when she was 6 months old that she had a hearing loss, I would have gotten her hearing aids right away," she says. "Once we got them, her personality changed overnight. Gone was the frustration, the exhaustion. The fatigue started to melt away. There was no more collapsing on the floor in a ball—she was just so much happier."

Becky went to the same preschool program as Elizabeth, though she was in a different class. Because of provincial regulations, Becky didn't qualify for an FM system until she was in kindergarten. Kathy wasn't thrilled with the device to begin with; she felt the FM made everything too loud. "When I would go up to some of the other kids with their FMs and speak to them, they didn't hear me at all, and I could hear what they were hearing," she says.

Before Becky started kindergarten, at the same neighborhood school as Elizabeth, Kathy began lobbying for the school's parent council to purchase an FM sound field system. Largely because of her efforts, by the time Elizabeth was in sixth grade, all but one classroom had an FM system. The teachers became FM fans because they could get the attention of all the students without having to strain their voices.

One reason Kathy put so much effort into arranging for the systems was that she didn't want Becky to stand out. "I've been through that, and I know what a singled out kid turns out like," she says. "It's really hard for them. Does Becky feel different? I don't think so—not yet, anyway. She hasn't expressed that to me. She's never expressed any kind of remorse or sadness or those kind of things although my other daughter, who wears leg braces, has said to me, 'When am I going to be able to run?' Things like that just break your heart because you know that this is not going to be. It's not going to happen. And that whole experience has definitely colored how I am treating this experience."

She's certainly passed on a sense of confidence. Not long ago two of Becky's classmates commented about how she doesn't hear well in French class and needs help. Becky retorted, "Yeah, but I *see* better than both of you."

When children ask why Becky has to wear hearing aids, Kathy likens them to glasses. "They're both aidable disabilities, as opposed to Elfi's, which is only partially aidable. She can't run, but Becky can play viola and go to dance class."

## Cochlear Implants for Carter

Not long after learning her son, Carter, was profoundly deaf, Cheri, who lived in North Carolina at the time, received a newsletter from the School for the Deaf in her area.

"They were spotlighting one of the students who had been named a shift manager at McDonald's," she recalls. "That's when it hit me—am I totally in denial?"

It wasn't that Cheri and her husband didn't appreciate that such a job "would be a huge feat for some children," she says. It's just that until that point, she'd been thinking about how Carter's deafness would affect his toddler years, his childhood, the foreseeable future. It hadn't occurred to her to consider how it might affect his entire life and that it could possibly limit his career options.

Six months of trial hearing aid use showed amplification to be of little benefit, so at 19 months Carter received a cochlear implant. Cheri and her husband knew the ideal scenario was for one of them to quit work to stay home to care for him, but that was not realistic for them. Instead, they kept their jobs and found a day care for Carter.

"We're not made out of money, so we need our income, plus for my sanity, I needed it more than anything, so that put another huge demand on me," Cheri says. "I felt that was going to take me over the edge. I felt that if anything fails, it will all be on my head, but looking back, it would not have worked out as good as it has if we had taken another route, because that day care center has been awesome."

At the day care center, Carter worked with an itinerant teacher and an inclusion specialist. At home his parents pointed out sounds, turned him to face them, and explained what they were. "It was like having a newborn baby," Cheri recalls.

By age 4, Carter was shushing his parents so he could concentrate on hitting a golf ball. By 6, in school, he was social, making friends, and impressing his teachers. But there were setbacks, the most traumatic of which occurred when the implant began failing after a year and Carter had to undergo surgery to replace it.

The next reality check came when the couple's third child, Hailey, who was born 2 years after Carter, failed her newborn hearing screening. Initially Cheri wasn't upset. "I guess because we had traveled down that road, we knew that life would go on."

Then came the shocking news: Hailey wasn't profoundly deaf; she had a severe-to-profound loss and would need hearing aids.

"We said, 'Well, what do we do now?'" Cheri says, "and the audiologist said it was almost as if we were disappointed she had hearing. I said no, it was just that we knew how to proceed if she was totally deaf."

Hailey did very well with her hearing aids, developing age-appropriate speech and language skills, and such acute hearing that one night, when Cheri began singing along with a lullaby on a CD player, Hailey said, "Shhhhh!"

But Hailey's hearing loss fluctuated. By the time she was 4, her language skills were beginning to plateau. Tests showed that she, too, was a candidate for an implant. "It helped her out tremendously," Cheri says. "Her speech is beautiful."

## A New Kind of Hearing Aid

Jesse was only minutes old when the doctor who delivered him in 1995 informed his parents that he had a hearing loss. She could tell from looking at his ears.

Jesse has microtia and atresia. Microtia is characterized by a small, abnormally shaped, or absent outer ear and atresia by the absence or incomplete formation of the ear canals. Jesse's ears are about two thirds of normal size. Instead of being open, his ear canals are filled with bone and tissue.

Jesse's mother, Teresa, is a speech-language pathologist who knew some sign language and had done a practicum with an agency that works with families of children who are deaf and hard of hearing. His dad, Steve, is an electronics engineer. The couple took a very workmanlike approach to their firstborn's hearing loss.

"We didn't go through the typical grief thing," Teresa says. "We had this huge background knowledge that was great. I knew all sorts of things about speech and language and signing. My husband covered everything we had to know about the technical end."

But a couple of weeks after Jesse was born, before Teresa and her husband had any confirmation that their son's loss had no sensorineural component, Teresa did shed a tear or two. "I was worrying that he might not enjoy music," she says.

As it turned out, Jesse's moderate-to-severe loss is purely conductive. "It's like plugging your ears totally efficiently," Teresa explains.

Jesse loves music, both playing and listening to it. He took a year of piano when he was 7 and began violin lessons at 8. He's now an avid fiddler, traveling up to 45 minutes on a weeknight to play with a fiddle group.

When he was 7, he began undergoing surgery to get a bone-anchored hearing aid (BAHA). It's made a big and positive difference in his hearing.

"I like the sound better," he says. "Somehow it sounds sharper and clearer."

It's also more practical for a boy who likes to move around. When Jesse was a baby, he used a headband to keep his hearing aids in place, but as he grew older he needed something less feminine. His audiologist had modified earmolds made for him. They kept the aids in, but Jesse still needed double-sided tape to hold the oscillator, or vibrating part of his bone conducting aid, in place. Every time he removed the oscillator or sweated even a bit, he had to change the tape. The BAHA is all one piece and it attaches to a screw that's been surgically implanted in Jesse's skull. As Teresa says, "You snap it into place and poof! It's on."

Jesse has always been a good listener, a function, his mother thinks, of his having been aided from birth. But the BAHA has certainly made things better.

Not long after Jesse got the BAHA, he went for a bike ride with his family. While waiting to cross the street, Jesse stopped and began looking carefully around him. "What are you looking for?" his father asked.

"I'm looking for the cricket," Jesse replied.

"He heard it," Teresa says, the wonder still fresh in her voice. "It was actually across the street. He hadn't been able to hear a cricket from that far away before."

## Uprooting The Family

Katy was hospitalized with meningitis at 15 months. Her parents, Dee Ann and Lee, left their two other children with relatives back home, 150 miles away, and stayed in a Ronald McDonald house during the 6 weeks it took Katy to recover. The illness destroyed her sense of balance and left her with no hearing in one ear and a severe-to-profound loss in the other. Doctors told the family she would never play sports, ride a bike, ski, swim, or read past a fifth grade level.

"Of course it was devastating news," Dee Ann says. "However, she was sick for so long, so we were very aware that the deafness was not the worst thing that could've happened."

Not long after the diagnosis, while Katy was still in the hospital, Dee Ann and Lee met the pastor of a local church, who was on an outing with a group of deaf teenagers.

"We nearly beat him down asking questions," Dee Ann says. "After a few minutes, he asked how to contact us later, and he said he would put together a group of parents for us to visit with. Two days later, we went to his house, and we became a little wary when we saw 10 other cars. We didn't want some overpowering religious indoctrination. But that was not what happened. The pastor had assembled parents of deaf kids who communicated in different ways, had made mistakes in their children's education, had successful educational experiences, who had vastly different opinions and experiences. We listened and questioned and talked with those wonderful people for about 4 hours. Then we began our pursuit of the best option available for our daughter."

After spending months investigating educational opportunities, Dee Ann and Lee decided the best option was a school in Omaha, 400 miles from their home. They packed up the family and moved.

"Katy's hearing loss impacted our family in a major way because our life had to change completely," Dee Ann says. "We had been ranchers in a rural area, and because no help was available there, we had to move and change every aspect of our lives. It was no longer possible to stay in the cattle business. We have developed a new business in an entirely different industry. It was maybe a little hard on the other children in the family, but they adjusted."

The move certainly benefited Katy. She got nearly all As in school, made the honor roll, played sports, played saxophone in the band, and has traveled as far as Japan on her own.

"She's not a great singer, but then, neither is anyone else in the family," Dee Ann says. "She actually did better in band than the other four kids, but ran out of time to practice because she wanted to be doing sports."

Katy attended a competitive liberal arts college in Iowa, where she captained the women's basketball team and made all-conference 4 years in a row. She became the second leading all-time scorer at the college. Now 24, she teaches school and coaches basketball in Arizona. You can read more about her in our last chapter, "Advice from the Trenches."

"The hardest thing for me is those rare moments when I ask myself, 'What if?'" Dee Ann says. "Katy has adapted so well, has had so many successes, that sometimes I forget about her constant struggle. But once, in a quiet moment when we were thinking about 'What if I could have one wish?' she wished she could hear. It made me so sad, because for her it is constant.

"I think, although she has a world of friends and is outgoing and well liked, it has impacted her socially. If she didn't have her sports, she would have struggled more to find her niche. She can't 'whisper' secrets like other girls do, she has to ask for clarification often, she misses out on parts of conversations. These are the kinds of things I grieve about in private. I do not dwell on them, but on occasion, I feel sad."

## Toby: Learning to Speak Made the Difference

"I knew in my heart that there was something very wrong when my son was 20 to 22 months old," says Vicki, who lives in Ottawa, Ontario. "He did not speak, but worse, he clearly usually did not understand."

During the week he turned 2, Toby was diagnosed with a moderate-to-severe bilateral sensorineural hearing loss. Two weeks later, Vicki and her husband, Glen, were invited to a meeting at the Children's Hospital of Eastern Ontario (CHEO), where Toby would receive his audiology care to the end of his teen years. They were invited to bring other relatives, and all four grandparents came. Also present were an audiologist, a social worker, and an auditory-verbal therapist (AVT).

Today, more than 25 years later, Vicki recalls that the meeting was vital to the family's understanding and acceptance of the diagnosis.

"CHEO has had a world-class AVT program for over 25 years," she says. "This program was explained to us on the day of the diagnosis, and quite honestly, I do not remember having other options explained to me, or that we ever seriously considered other options. We did have an acquaintance in our neighborhood who tried very hard to talk us into signing, but I never took her seriously because I couldn't really understand why we would do that when the other option seemed to make so much sense. She is the hearing daughter of signing deaf parents, and has always been and continues to be a very strong advocate for that community. But we were a hearing, speaking family, with one other son. It was just obvious to us that we would at least try speech—and why shouldn't it work?"

It did work. "Now that we know a great deal more about the choices, we are even more convinced that we made the right choice for our son," Vicki says. "Anything else for that child would have been a travesty. And furthermore, he tells us regularly that he is delighted that we made the choice we did, and that he cannot imagine being anything other than oral."

Toby developed into an avid athlete—he skateboards and plays hockey, baseball, and soccer. Because he doesn't use the FM during sports, he, his coaches, and teammates developed other strategies, among them yelling and using hand signals.

An extrovert, he also makes friends easily. Now 28 and working at a Toronto television station, he's a great source of pride to his parents. You will read more about him in the last chapter.

"Our son is a fine young man who loves his work and who has good social and communication skills," his mother says. "We had many challenges along the way—what parent does not? When one looks at the pain, suffering, illness, grief, and unhappiness in the lives of so many, even most, what is moderate-to-severe hearing loss? Not such a big deal.

"Having said that, as long as I live, mostly at times when I least expect it, I will get a huge lump in my throat that our son is deaf and that he has to deal with this," she says. "This is not how we 'ordered' him, but that is how he came, and we are probably all better people for it. But I tell you, I cried throughout his college graduation ceremony!"

# 9

# ADVOCATING FOR YOUR CHILD

Before I began researching this chapter, my concept of advocacy was telling people on the playground, in school, social activities, or any new situation that Elizabeth has a hearing loss. It was making clear that even though she wears hearing aids, she still doesn't hear as well as someone with normal hearing. Whoever is speaking will have to accommodate. Generally, that will involve facing her, speaking clearly or loudly—shouting isn't necessary but whispering is unacceptable—and checking to make sure she has understood what's been said.

After talking to parents and experts who had to battle for their children's rights and needs, I alternated between feeling embarrassed about my naiveté and grateful that things had gone so easily for Elizabeth that I'd been able to labor under my illusions for so long. At the same time, I came to understand that whether someone's efforts are as minor as a one-time request to an education specialist or as extreme as having to hire a lawyer for a court hearing, at its very basic level, advocacy is what I'd assumed from the beginning: it means doing what is necessary to make sure our children are treated fairly and afforded the same opportunities as their normal-hearing peers, whether on the playground, in school, at public gatherings, or by their health care providers.

Whether you realize it or not, you have already advocated for your child. Every time you take him to the audiologist because his earmolds don't seem to be fitting or the volume control on his hearing aids isn't functioning, you're advocating. Every time you've reminded the soccer coach that he has to turn on the FM before he addresses your daughter's team, every time you've asked a teenager behind a fast food counter to repeat her question because your daughter, who wears hearing aids, doesn't hear well in crowded, noisy places, you've been an advocate.

Too many of us are misled into assuming advocacy is always a complicated process that requires lawyers, judges, professional experts, and years of legal battles. For some parents, sadly, that is the case. For more of us, I hope, advocacy will be a simpler, more direct process. For all of us with young children, it's something we'll likely deal with on some level every day, largely because our children don't always know when and how to speak up for themselves. One of the most important lessons we must teach them is how to do just that.

I'm usually quite confident and comfortable speaking up for what I believe in, largely because I've always felt my concerns are taken seriously. But when it came to acting as an advocate for Elizabeth, especially in the early days of her diagnosis, I was unpleasantly surprised to discover how often people didn't seem to hear what I was saying. The new teacher in Elizabeth's Kindermusik class insisted on speaking in a whisper even though I told her repeatedly that Elizabeth couldn't hear unless she spoke up. The gymnastics teacher, whom I had just reminded about Elizabeth's diagnosis, looked me straight in the eye and said, in all seriousness, "Oh, I think she can hear. I think she's just not paying attention."

At first I blamed myself: I wasn't convincing enough because I was having such a hard time accepting Elizabeth's hearing loss. But after talking to parents who had similar experiences and, more importantly, after dealing with people who did take my concerns seriously, I began to see there is no one way to advocate: different situations call for different approaches. Some people refuse to be convinced; others seem to listen with rapt attention and then proceed as if they didn't comprehend a word you said. Others, bless their hearts, do exactly as you ask. My job—any parent's job—is to learn to deal with each situation to make sure my child can hear and understand.

Unless Elizabeth has her hair pulled back so her hearing aids are visible, people meeting her have no idea she has a hearing loss. Sometimes even when her hair is pulled back and her hearing aids are visible, people don't notice. For the first few years after she began wearing hearing aids, whenever a stranger would say something to her in a crowded, noisy place and she didn't respond, I'd feel obligated to explain about the hearing loss. By the time she was 8, I was more likely to give her a chance to explain it herself. If she didn't, or if she seemed uncomfortable, I'd say something. But as she grew older, I began to sense that it was intrusive and unnecessary for me to speak for her, and that it was up to her to decide when she wanted to bring it up and to whom.

Some children are comfortable advocating for themselves at a young age. Others aren't, says Diane Schmidt, who has spoken to many parents as part of her job as Supervisor of the Media/Graphics Department at Boys Town National Research Hospital in Omaha, NE, where she helped put together the excellent Web site, http://www.babyhearing.org.

"I think Mom and Dad should be helping out in one way or another all the time, by which I mean you observe and step in when needed," Diane says. "If the child is handling the situation easily on their own, leave them alone. If they're struggling or shy, or the other person isn't responding well to them, step in and help. Most kids are really good at letting you know when they need a little help, whether it be by telling you or by a look or their body language. I think we just need to follow their lead."

If you're in a situation where your child needs to know everything that's going on, you may have to step in, even if your child feels he's in control. But it's also important to remember that sometimes we cause more problems and embarrassment by jumping in when our kids are confident they're handling everything. If you're finding that's happening on a regular basis, it's best to have a talk with your child in private, to explain why you feel the need to step in, and also to find out what he feels would work better.

Diane's daughter, Christin, who is now an adult with a family of her own, is profoundly deaf. From the day Christin started school in a mainstream program, Diane talked to her about her rights in terms she could understand. Diane would frequently ask Christin how things were going with her interpreter, whether she could understand her clearly, if the interpreter was the one disciplining her in class if she wasn't paying attention (which was forbidden), and if the interpreter was interpreting everything the other children were saying. If there was any doubt, Diane would remind her that it was her right to have an interpreter she could clearly under-stand and who was interpreting everything being said in the class-room. She'd encourage Christin to speak to the teacher of the deaf at the school, and she'd follow up in a few days by asking if Christin had done that.

"I didn't usually ask her to talk to the interpreter directly, because often they don't feel like a child has the right to tell them what to do or not to do, and the child goes away feeling that they shouldn't have said anything," Diane says.

If Christin hadn't talked to the teacher or was hesitant about doing so, Diane would offer to do it herself. Christin often preferred that option when she was younger. As she grew older and more confident, she'd sometimes speak to the teacher about a problem first, and then tell her mother.

When Christin was in middle school, she and her fellow deaf and hard-of-hearing classmates had an incompetent interpreter. The stu-dents couldn't understand her, and her behavior was unacceptable. Among other things, she'd sit cross-legged on top of a desk in front of her male junior high school students. The resource teacher for deaf students called Diane to ask if she would come into the school to observe the interpreter. The teacher said she had a gut feeling the woman wasn't qualified, and the administration responded better to parental concerns than to complaints from teachers.

Before Diane had a chance to speak to the resource teacher again, Christin came home and announced that she and her class-mates had met and were going to bring their complaints to the teacher themselves. As a result of their efforts and parental com-plaints, the interpreter was removed, put on probation, and told she'd have to attend remedial signing classes consistently for a year.

When the special education director called Diane to explain the situation, Diane said she would not accept the interpreter work-ing with Christin again, regardless of how much additional training she had.

"We had a rather heated discussion on this, but I insisted my child would not be the guinea pig during this interpreter's proba-tion period," Diane says. "In the end, Christin never had her again, and before long, she was gone. But this is an example of how our kids can learn to advocate for themselves, which I think is our goal from day one. They need guidance and lots of support to do it, but they can and do learn how."

## The Basics of Advocacy

Whether you're attempting to convince the cafeteria director to serve spinach for lunch every day or trying to secure preferential seating for your hard-of-hearing child in the classroom, the basics of advocacy are the same: start with the source. Just as you wouldn't go to the food supplier to complain about the lunch menu, your first step in advocating for your child in the classroom shouldn't be to make an appointment with the superintendent or the head of the school board.

Get to know your child's teachers. Perhaps they've had experience with hard-of-hearing children. If they haven't, make an appointment to sit down with them and explain your child's needs. Offer literature. For me one of the most helpful books available was the third edition of *Our Forgotten Children: Hard of Hearing Pupils in the Public Schools*, edited by Julia Davis, PhD, and published by Self Help for Hard of Hearing People (see Recommended Readings).

Many school districts have audiologists who are salaried employees; others are on contract to serve school-age children. As a group, *educational audiologists* are a special breed. They enjoy working in the educational environment and are often great advocates for kids and families. They often provide a vital link between the medical center audiologists and the intervention setting. The Web site for the Educational Audiology Association (http://www.edaud.org), although designed primarily for professionals, has links of interest to parents and also a directory of educational audiologists in the United States.

In the United States, children with special needs up to the age of 21 are protected by the Individuals with Disabilities Education Improvement Act (IDEA), which guarantees that all children with disabilities who are in need of special education have access to "a free appropriate public education which emphasizes special education and related services designed to meet their unique needs" (U.S. Department of Education, 2004; see Info Box).

To receive federal funds under IDEA, each state must have an educational plan that complies with the law's standards and procedures. Although the most significant features will be consistent, states vary in their procedural requirements. Your local education agency or state Department of Public Instruction can provide you with information about IDEA requirements for your state.

## The Individuals with Disabilities
## Education Improvement Act

*In the United States, children who require special education and related services may be classified as educationally disabled and subsequently protected under the Individuals with Disabilities Education Improvement Act (IDEA[1]). Children with hearing loss fall into this category, usually under the deaf and hard of hearing eligibility classification. IDEA has a process to determine eligibility and the need for special education and related services.*

*Children 3 and older who are eligible for services are required to have an individualized education program (IEP), which documents how a school district must meet their educational needs. Those under the age of 3 are required to have an individualized family service plan (IFSP), which documents and guides the early intervention process for them and their families.*

*The lead agency is responsible for administering the infant and toddler program depends on the state where you live. Your local school officials will be able to refer you to the proper agency.*

*An excellent resource for learning more about your child's rights is:* IDEA Advocacy for Children Who Are Deaf or Hard of Hearing, *by Bonnie Poitras Tucker (1997).*

In Canada, federal disability laws are broader and scattered under several pieces of legislation, the most prominent being the Charter of Rights and Freedoms. Because education falls under provincial jurisdiction, the best way to learn your child's rights is to check with the Department of Education in your province or territory.

In the United States, if your child is being considered for special services you will be scheduled for a multidisciplinary team evaluation. Assuming your child meets eligibility criteria, the team will work with you to develop an individualized family service plan (IFSP) if your child is younger than 3. For children 3 and older, the plan is called an individualized education plan (IEP; see Info Box).

---

[1]The word "improvement" was added in 2004 but most people still call it IDEA.

## The Individualized Education Plan (IEP): Important Points to Remember

■ *You do not have to sign an IEP that has been prepared by a teacher before the IEP meeting if you do not agree with its content. The purpose of the meeting is to determine the best educational placement for your child. A committee is convened for that purpose.*

■ *You have the right to request that the IEP committee be reconvened if you do not believe that the IEP is working.*

■ *You have the right to bring outside support people to the IEP meeting. You can request that an advocate, your child's private psychologist, psychiatrist, or any other person attend the meeting.*

■ *The best way to resolve conflicts is through mediation. Overtly expressed anger raises defenses at a meeting and rarely results in the changes you want. A "squeaky wheel" that keeps requesting needed accommodations in a friendly manner will be heard over the angry outburst. Be consistent and work through to achieve needed educational programs.*

■ *If the IEP team leader says that the meeting can only last for a period of time and requests that you sign the IEP document even though you do not believe the process has been completed, request that the committee reconvene at a different time to complete the process.*

■ *Stay involved. If the IEP is written at the end of the school year, make certain it is being implemented at the beginning of the next school year. This is especially important at times of transition. A child who leaves elementary school to begin middle school may find that teachers have not been made adequately aware of needed accommodations. Follow through to see that they are put into place.*

■ *Be sure that accommodations requested are reasonable within the context of the program. For example, it may not be possible for the teacher to rewrite a test. In such cases, ask instead if there are other tests that can measure the*

> *same thing or accommodations that can better enable the student to take the test.*
>
> ■ *For older children, IEP regulations encourage student participation in the process. School officials are required to invite students 16 years and older to attend the transitional IEP meeting.*
>
> ■ *Finally, if an IEP meeting is set at a time when you cannot attend, request a time when you will be able to attend.*
>
> Excerpted from "Understanding the IEP Process," LD OnLine. Available from http://www.ldonline.org/indepth/iep. Used with permission.

The IEP, which is required only in public schools in the United States and which is a legal document, will follow your child through his school years, with updates and revisions as needed. See Resources for additional resources that describe the IFSP, IEP, and the legal rights of families (also see Info Box).

In Canada, the rights of individuals with disabilities are outlined in the Charter of Rights and Freedoms, but the accommodations your child will receive will depend on where you live and where he goes to school. Most school districts will have a document similar in style to that of the IEP, although it is not considered a legal document. Like its U.S. counterpart, it is designed to identify your child's educational needs and how the school will meet them in a given year. The plan should be examined and revised at least once a year, or more often if necessary.

It seems straightforward enough, but conflicts do arise. You may not agree with what the school is offering your child, and the school may not agree with what you believe your child needs. If that happens, the best approach is a nonconfrontational one. Provide evidence to back your claims, either in the form of studies or research or letters from your child's audiologist, speech-language pathologist (SLP), teacher of the deaf and hard of hearing, or other appropriate specialists. Perhaps the school officials truly are adversarial, but there are good reasons not to lose your temper and start threatening the first time someone disagrees with you. Losing control is unprofessional and gives people a reason not to take you seriously. It also keeps you from focusing on the important task, which is to ensure that your child gets a solid education.

## Understanding Your Legal Rights

*In United States, the Individuals with Disabilities Education Improvement Act (IDEA) is the federal law that ensures a "free appropriate public education" to children with disabilities. This means that children who qualify under IDEA are eligible for the specialized instruction and support services necessary for their educational needs in a "least restrictive" environment; that is, in an environment where education is provided, to the extent possible, with children who do not have disabilities. Section 504 of the Rehabilitation Act of 1973 protects the rights of people with disabilities of all ages in programs and activities that receive federal funds. It states that a person with a disability cannot, because of the disability, be excluded from participation in, denied benefits of, or subjected to discrimination under a program that receives federal funding. Accordingly, school districts are required to provide a "free and appropriate public education" to each child who qualifies, regardless of the nature or severity of the disability.*

*What does this mean for children with hearing loss and how does Section 504 of the Rehabilitation Act differ from IDEA? First, Section 504 is part of a civil rights law. In contrast, IDEA is an educational law. To qualify for an IEP under IDEA, a child must demonstrate the need for specialized instruction, that is, a special education program that is different from what is typically provided. If a child can learn from the regular education curriculum and does not qualify for special education, a 504 plan may be appropriate. Children with IEPs may qualify for services under Section 504, but those who do not qualify for an IEP will need to have their 504 plans developed separately.*

*School districts in the United States have a legal obligation to identify children with disabilities and provide for their needs, but your advocacy and assistance may be necessary. Children with hearing loss who show evidence of developmental delays generally have no difficulty qualifying for an IEP. But those who were identified early and who received appropriate services may begin their school years without developmental delays. For those children, a 504 plan can help ensure access to the accommodations needed for full participation in the classroom.*

## Know Who You're Dealing With

Bruce Goldstein is a Buffalo, NY, lawyer, whose specialization in disability law arose out of personal need. His two daughters were born deaf, and when they were getting ready to start school in the late 1970s, Bruce and his wife did extensive research to figure out where their children could get the best public education. The Individuals with Disabilities Education Act (which has since been reauthorized as the Individuals with Disabilities Education Improvement Act) had been in effect since 1976, the year the younger Goldstein daughter was born. "That's how I got into this law—I began investigating for them," Bruce says.

Since then, he has become a highly respected expert, sought after by both parents and school districts throughout North America. Some of his cases have set state and national precedent in disability law. His observations about advocacy in the education arena are insightful and valuable to all parents.

"You have to know who you're dealing with," he says. "In some school districts, you've got special ed directors who are child friendly, if you will, and then you've got others who are pure bureaucratic types. So you've got to try, as you would in any other situation where you're trying to persuade someone, to use some empathy and put yourself in the shoes of the other person. If you're dealing with a child-friendly person, you'd talk about the child and the importance of the child's progress. If you're dealing with a bureaucratic type, you want to emphasize that it's not going to cost much more, or cost anything more at all."

There are times when no matter how reasonable one party is, an impasse is inevitable. It may sound overly simple to say the world is made up of "good" school districts and "bad" school districts, but sometimes that's how it seems, says Bruce, who adds that there are also plenty of shades of gray.

"The 'bad' districts will be operating the way they are either because they're trying to save money or out of ignorance or out of understaffing, so they'd have to do things in an assembly line fashion," he says. "They aren't prepared to give each child the time that is necessary, or they might be dealing out of ego or fighting over control with the parent, or they may just be working out of inertia."

By the same token, Bruce adds, there are parents who develop a reputation for being difficult, "so from the school district's side, nothing you're going to do is going to satisfy them."

My husband would be the first person to tell you I'm opinionated and insist on doing everything my way. At home, maybe. But he never saw me approach the principal at Elizabeth's elementary school. When Elizabeth was in first grade, the school receptionist, Jan, whose own daughter has a hearing loss similar to Elizabeth's, told me to ask the principal if the school would pay for Elizabeth's FM batteries and repairs.

"She uses the FM for school," Jan told me. "We should be paying for the batteries and repairs."

I was skeptical and didn't want to look greedy, but after thinking about it for a few days, I asked Robin, the principal. "Fine," she said to me, and for the next year and a half, I submitted bills for every package of AA batteries I bought for the FM and every repair. Then one day, Jan told me that the budget was tight, so the school could no longer afford the expense. No problem, I said. We'd just go back to paying, and claiming the cost on our income tax.

Not long after that, we learned Elizabeth needed a new FM. Rhiannon, one of her audiologists, said the school should pay for it. "I'll call your principal," she said.

My chest tightened. "The school doesn't have enough money," I told her. If they couldn't afford a few hundred dollars for repairs and batteries, where were they going to find the $3,000 for a new FM?

"They can pay for it," Rhiannon said. "They receive extra money because of Elizabeth's hearing loss, and this is one of the things it's for. Don't worry. I'll take care of it."

I went home and had a long talk with Dave. His supplemental health insurance provided us with a 5-year $1000 allowance for hearing aids and related expenses. We'd blown that 4 years earlier, paying for Elizabeth's first hearing aids and her FM. In fact, we'd gone well over the budget and had paid for some of the equipment out of pocket. If necessary, we could have scraped together money for a new FM system, but if we waited another year, the health insurance would kick back in and it would be covered. But could we wait another year? The FM system seemed to break down every few months, and nearly every day I found myself having to press the boots to the hearing aids to guarantee a connection or to fiddle with the antenna rings to avoid static.

The next day I went to the principal's office and said if the school couldn't afford the FM, Dave and I would find a way to pay for it. "Don't worry about it, Debby," Robin assured me. "We'll make it work. This is our responsibility, and we'll handle it."

When she called me into her office after hearing from Rhiannon and asked whether it would be okay to buy the less expensive FM, the one with wires instead of the more discreet wireless version Elizabeth was comfortable with, I balked. Sure, it was more economical, but I knew from talking to other parents and audiologists that it was also much less desirable for a child who would rather not call extra attention to herself.

"No," I said. "She really needs the wireless, with the boots that don't have the rings attached. The one with the rings just isn't durable enough."

A week later, Elizabeth had the newest FM available. But there was a catch: Robin wanted it left at school when Elizabeth wasn't using it. Unlike the FM we'd gotten when Elizabeth was 3, this one belonged to the school, and we couldn't use it at violin lessons, soccer, Hebrew school, or on vacations. I could understand that, but I still wanted it at home: otherwise I'd have to do two equipment checks every day, one at home, and then at school. Plus, it would mean having to take Elizabeth's aids off when she got to school to put the FM boots on, which would be time consuming and, undoubtedly, annoying for both her and for me.

Peter, another of Elizabeth's audiologists, recommended that not only should we keep the FM at our house, we should be able to use it at our discretion. He told me about other families who used their school-owned FMs for non-school events.

"Learning doesn't take place just between school hours," he reminded me.

He was right—I knew he was. But we had our own FM, fragile and aging though it was. I couldn't bring myself to insist that Robin let us use the new one just because it was new and in better condition. Sure, Elizabeth might have been entitled to use it during non-school hours, but was it right to argue for something just because I could, not because she actually needed it? In the end, I decided, for me, it wasn't. However, I did tell Robin we needed to keep the FM at our house so I could do daily equipment checks, but that we wouldn't use it for anything other than school. She agreed without hesitation.

A year later, when I talked to Bruce Goldstein, I felt more validated in that decision. "Sometimes you have to look at the big picture and not try to get every little thing you might think you're entitled to," he told me. "When my daughters were going through the public school system, there were a number of occasions when my wife and I were aware the district wasn't implementing the IEP to the full extent, but on a number of occasions we didn't say anything because the more important thing was to keep good relations and make sure that things generally were being done properly. Look at anything in life, and how often is it really being done 100% to the hilt? So you look for substantially what's needed, rather than going for every last little item. You pick your fights."

Even though Bruce is a lawyer, a courtroom is his last choice as a venue for settling disputes. At least 95% of the time, he and his colleagues are able to settle a case without going to a hearing. "There are lots of different ways you can accomplish your goals, as long as you're practical in how you deal with it," he says.

## A Mother Takes Her Fight to the State Stage

The best advice I've seen on how to conduct a dignified and successful advocacy campaign comes from Trish Freeman, a Kentucky mother who had to battle her insurance company before it would agree to pay for hearing aids for her two sons. When Trish's oldest son was 3 and her youngest 2 years old, they were diagnosed with mild and moderate losses, respectively. The losses turned out to be progressive, and the family had to buy new hearing aids at a rate of a pair a year. Within 4 years, both boys were profoundly deaf and the family found itself having to pay for its fourth pair of aids in as many years.

Until then, Trish says, she'd accepted her HMO's policy of not paying for hearing aids. "When it came time for the fourth one," she recalls, "I said, enough of this already. This is not right. We have this condition and it's affecting their health. I kept telling myself that if they were disabled because they had a physical disability, like a club foot, the insurance company would be paying for surgery, but they're not going to pay for children who can't hear? What's the difference? It's an arbitrary distinction they've made."

The HMO's rationale was that hearing aids aren't medically necessary. As a representative explained to Trish, the HMO considered hearing aids "life-enhancing services" and therefore not eligible for coverage.

For 8 months, Trish wrote detailed, articulate letters to the HMO. She cited studies and evidence from the company's own certificate of coverage to highlight the flaws in its logic. Each appeal was turned down. Convincing the insurance company was beginning to look hopeless, but Trish couldn't bring herself to quit. The final step was a grievance hearing, and she was determined to have her say there.

Weeks went by and Trish hadn't heard from the company, so she called and asked the receptionist the date of the hearing. "You can't come," the receptionist informed her. "The committee will meet and they will review what you submit."

Trish was furious. "A hearing means your case will be heard, that you'll be able to present your case, not that you submit your documents in writing," she says. "I told the receptionist, 'You need to look up your definition of the word *hearing* and if you don't intend people to come, you need to change the language in your certificate of coverage.'"

The receptionist spoke to the HMO's medical director, who made an exception and allowed Trish to attend the hearing. There, Trish spoke passionately about her sons' hearing loss and why her older son needed a new pair of sophisticated digital aids that would transpose the high-frequency sounds that he could barely hear into lower frequencies that he could. The committee—a pediatrician, an ENT, the medical director, and other physicians—listened quietly.

"Not a single one of them asked me a question," she says. "They all sat there looking at me with condescending looks on their faces, as if they were thinking, 'Oh, you poor thing.' They just smiled at me and shook their heads and said, 'Thank you. You can go now.' I was dismissed. I didn't get to hear any of their discussions. I went home and promptly had a big glass of wine and told my husband, 'We'll still be paying for the hearing aids, but at least I tried.'"

Trish guessed wrong: a week later, the HMO sent her a letter saying they'd pay for the aids. But happy as she was with her victory, Trish was also still reeling from the experience. "It was an eye opener to the whole process," she says.

A pharmacist with a PhD in pharmacology, Trish is the director of professional practice programs at the University of Kentucky College of Pharmacy. She knows science, and she's accustomed to dealing with bureaucracies. But her 8-month struggle with her HMO over her sons' hearing aids, a struggle she waged without any legal help, nearly wore her down.

"Here I am, a health care professional. I have all these skills, and yet it was a daunting task for me," she says. Her biggest support came from the Internet, specifically a site called Listen-Up (http://www .listen-up.org), which offers advice and template letters, including now her own, for parents in similar situations.

"I thought, other parents who are facing this situation, the majority of them are not likely to have the same skill set, and if it was a daunting task for me, imagine what it would be like for them. Most people would have just thrown their hands up—they would have said, 'This is impossible.' And that's not right. Other parents shouldn't have to go through this to get the services they need for their children."

When the opportunity to help those parents presented itself, Trish was ready. One night not long after the battle with the HMO had come to a successful conclusion, she picked up the latest issue of *Volta Voices*, the monthly magazine of the Alexander Graham Bell Association for the Deaf and Hard of Hearing (AG Bell Association), one of the world's largest membership organizations and information centers on hearing loss. Her intent was to flip through the magazine before she fell asleep, but an article caught her attention and wouldn't let go. It was by a Maryland mother who was working to convince her state legislature to pass a law requiring insurance companies to cover hearing aids.

*Somebody ought to do that in Kentucky*, Trish thought to herself. And a little while later, after she'd turned off the light but still couldn't sleep, she decided she would be that somebody. "I had never even contemplated anything like that before, but all of a sudden I was motivated and empowered," she says.

She climbed out of bed that instant and drafted e-mails to the man who had written the article and to the child advocate at the AG Bell Association. The next day, the two wrote back advising Trish to find a sponsor in the state legislature. A lifelong Kentuckian, she contacted Sen. Vernie McGaha, who had been elected 3 years earlier. Sen. McGaha happened to have been Trish's high school band director and principal at the junior high while her mother was principal at the high school.

Not everyone is likely to have such connections, but it's important to remember that legislators are elected to serve constituents. Even if you don't know a legislator personally, you should be able to approach one. You can get a list of your representatives from your state or provincial legislature. Use e-mail, the phone, or the postal service to contact those who have an interest in disabilities or special education or, if you have the time and energy, contact them all, until you find someone willing to take on your cause.

The AG Bell Association had sent Trish copies of the bills from Maryland and other states. She presented those to the senator. The bill they drafted was passed in the state senate and made it out of the house committee, but the session ended before the house could vote on it. Ultimately, Trish says, "it was a blessing in disguise" because it gave her the time she needed to build a strong grassroots campaign.

A member of the Kentucky State Commission for the Deaf and Hard of Hearing, Trish sought representatives from every sector in the deaf and hard-of-hearing community to serve on the study committee that would draft the new version of the bill: interpreters, vocational rehabilitation specialists, teachers of the hearing impaired, audiologists, parents, people who signed, the local AG Bell chapter. The idea was to cover every sector so each representative could be the contact person in his personal or professional community when it came time to generate support that would be needed to pass the bill.

The plan worked wonderfully. The 12 committee members met every few months and kept in touch mostly through e-mail. The first time they met in person was to fine-tune the language of the bill. They agreed that insurance companies should provide coverage for one hearing aid per impaired ear every 36 months, to a maximum of $1800 per ear, up until the age of 18. They also wanted the law to require companies to pay for related services, such as earmolds and fitting fees.

The e-mail network proved invaluable. If one of the legislators heard that a fellow house or senate member had a problem with the bill, Trish would be notified, and she in turn would send a broadcast e-mail to the study committee. Phones "would literally start ringing within minutes of my original e-mail broadcast," Trish says. "It really was amazing to see it in action."

As the date of the vote drew closer, the committee's publicity machine geared up. Members provided flyers, sample letters, talking points, and newsletter articles for meetings at schools and appropriate organizations throughout the state. They encouraged interested parties to write letters to their newspapers supporting the bill. Trish contacted the media to drum up further interest. Capitalizing on the state's early childhood initiative campaign, Education Pays, the committee came up with its own slogan, "Education should pay for all children, not just those with normal hearing!" which it repeated in letters to the media and legislators, and in flyers.

Among the people the committee invited to address the legislators were a mother whose child was diagnosed at birth a month after Kentucky implemented a newborn hearing screening act, and a 15-year-old hard-of-hearing high school student with a 4.0 GPA who was active in sports. Although the mother of the baby testified to her dismay at learning her child needed hearing aids and her insurance wouldn't pay for them, the 15-year-old boy had a happier story: through work, his family had insurance that did pay for hearing aids. He was able to provide firsthand evidence that coverage had benefits that were academic, athletic, and social.

Senate Bill 152 passed on March 22, 2002, a year and a half after Trish had first contacted Sen. McGaha. It went into effect on July 15, 2002. Ironically, the bill has no effect on the Freeman family: both Trish's sons now have cochlear implants, which were automatically covered by her HMO.

But she wouldn't have traded the experience, both for the opportunity to help other parents and for the chance to gain more insight into how childhood hearing loss is viewed by those who have no close experience with the condition.

"A lot of the stance of the medical community and insurance community is based on ignorance," she says. "They just don't have a clue, and it's our job to educate them about the negative outcomes: the negative health and social outcomes associated with improperly managed hearing impairment. Put some earplugs in and spend the day struggling to hear and struggling to communicate, and then see how you really feel about it." Joni Alberg, Executive Director of

Beginnings for Parents of Deaf and Hard of Hearing Children in Raleigh, NC, and a seasoned advocate for families, agrees. "Decision-makers must be informed about the needs of children with hearing loss. Who better to provide this education than parents? Or, even better, the children themselves. When decision-makers understand an issue, many are willing to act."

## Taking the School District to Court

If everybody was willing to accept proven facts and respond accordingly, advocacy would be a smooth process and disability lawyers would be out of a job. But it's not only the medical and insurance companies that often operate out of ignorance. Sometimes, as Alicia, a California mother of three, learned the hard way, it's the very people who are supposed to be educating our children.

Alicia had a 2-year-old son and a 3-year-old daughter when her third child, a daughter, Sylvia, was born in 2001. When Sylvia was 10 weeks old, she was diagnosed as profoundly deaf. Under IDEA, she was eligible for special services through her Special Education Local Plan Area, or SELPA. Had she been over 3 years old, the services would have been provided through the local school district.

By the time the SELPA specialists arrived for their evaluations when Sylvia was 3½ months old, Alicia and her husband had done enough research to know they wanted to raise her in an exclusively oral environment and arrange for her to have a cochlear implant when she was a year old.

"If Sylvia was our only daughter, then maybe we could move to a deaf community and really embrace signing and do all of these things, but she's not our only child, and we have to take everybody into account," Alicia says. "We honestly made a full-on effort to learn about signing, to learn about all the different methods, to make sure what we were thinking we wanted to do actually was what we wanted to do."

That's why it was especially frustrating for Alicia and her husband to see that the SELPA specialists weren't providing Sylvia with the kind of services they felt she needed. The teacher of the deaf and hard of hearing had Alicia put her daughter's hand on her throat to feel the vibration when she spoke. In Alicia's opinion, that was both outdated and inappropriate. "It wasn't an auditory method," she says. "She didn't mean to do it—it was natural for her, because that's what she's used to. But it just wasn't a match."

The SLP was used to working with children who had far less severe losses than Sylvia, children whose problems included stuttering and other speech disorders. She had very little experience with children who had or were about to have cochlear implants. Meanwhile, Alicia was taking classes at the John Tracy Clinic, a highly respected Los Angeles center that helps families with young children who are deaf and hard of hearing. The contrast between what she was learning there about what Sylvia needed to reach her potential and the services Sylvia was receiving at home made her even more determined to find suitable specialists.

As Sylvia approached her first birthday, Alicia found a local program she felt would meet her daughter's needs. She and her husband met with the SELPA authorities to explain why they felt the program was more appropriate, but the SELPA wouldn't pay. It insisted that its program, staffed by trained and accredited professionals, was sufficient.

Alicia and her husband continued to meet with the SELPA authorities. "When they said they weren't going to pay, I asked again," she says. "You need to try to compromise, you need to try to come up with creative solutions that work for everybody or do whatever you can and try to work it out, because going to a hearing is not fun, and not good for anybody. That's the last resort. It's expensive, it's very emotionally taxing and draining, and it's hard on everybody and it creates more work for everybody—mother, school district, everybody."

In the end, Alicia and her husband felt they had no choice. "If you really see no other way, if there's nowhere else to go and in your heart of hearts you know what they're giving you isn't good enough, or right, and that's what you need to do, then that's what you need to do. It comes down to how strong a parent are you, and how strong of an advocate are you for your child? How much can you stomach, and how much does your child need whatever it is you're asking for. It's a scale, and you have to just balance it and see which one tips up, and which one tips down."

After several unsuccessful meetings with the SELPA, Alicia and her husband decided they needed a lawyer. They contacted a local attorney and the AG Bell Association, which has a commitment to helping establish legal precedents for the rights of children who are deaf and hard of hearing and use spoken language. To that end, it will sometimes provide a lawyer for cases such as Alicia's. The Association asked Bruce Goldstein to represent the family. Bruce filed a motion for a hearing.

The hearing was split into two sessions, each lasting less than a week, but the process from the time Bruce and his partner got involved lasted several months. In the end, the administrative law judge agreed with Alicia and her husband that the program offered by the SELPA was not appropriate and the one the family had found was. And yet despite her "victory," Alicia still feels a loss.

"After the court case is over and you still have to work with the school district for another 12 years, you're not starting off on a real good foot," she says. "Once the court case is over, that doesn't mean you're not working with them anymore, it just means you've created animosity."

It's doubtful a school district or SELPA will try to retaliate against a family that's won a lawsuit, Bruce says. For one thing, it's illegal. For another, school districts are aware that parents who have won at a hearing may use that venue again. "I've found generally that school districts are more agreeable if they've lost a hearing, just because they want to avoid any future hearings."

Cases such as Alicia's, where the focus is on the qualifications of the professionals, are more likely to stir up negative feelings than are, say, cases where parents are simply trying to get services for their children. "If you're attacking people's credentials or qualifications, that tends to be taken a little more personally," Bruce says.

So what does he recommend for parents who feel they've alienated their children's future educators long before the first day of kindergarten? Strive for the high ground, he advises. Try to keep emotion out of it. Once the hearing is over, "go back and do what's in the child's best interest in recognition that the district and the family are going to have to live together for some time."

Alicia's plan is to tread lightly, to choose her battles carefully. "I'm just going to have to work really hard to try to mend a bridge," she says. "I don't have a choice. I've got three kids going through the school district, and two are in the special ed system."

# Know Your Rights, and Be Willing to Stand Up for Them

Corey and Sharon didn't have any children in the public school system when they began advocating for their first child, Regan, who had gotten a cochlear implant at 22 months. At age 3 she was working with an auditory-verbal (AV) therapist, and her parents wanted to send her to preschool with normal-hearing children to reinforce her language skills and prepare her for kindergarten. But when they approached the local school district, they were told that the district SLP, who had no experience with deaf children, would be working with their daughter. The SLP also told Corey and Sharon that Regan would be placed in the "integrated preschool program," where her classmates would have a variety of disabilities, including autism, dyslexia, multiple sclerosis, and speech impediments. There would be some "typical" children, to act as peers and mentors.

Corey and Sharon were determined that Regan attend a mainstream school. Equally important, they did not want to stop her AV therapy, which they knew was giving her the skills and language development she'd missed out on before she'd started wearing hearing aids after being diagnosed when she was a year old. But they couldn't convince the local authorities. Neither could Regan's AV therapist.

The attitude was "we're the school district, we know what's best for your child," Sharon recalls. "But they had never had a deaf kid before, or an implanted child. We were saying 'She's not a typical child with a language delay. She's a deaf child. We chose an approach for her to be rehabilitated. She needs to be in a regular preschool with regular kids, and she needs to be continuing with the therapy.'"

After Regan's AV therapist failed to convince the school district, he suggested the family involve a lawyer, and he put them in touch with AG Bell.

"We were scared to death," Sharon recalls. "We just thought, 'Oh my God, here we are, new parents, we've never dealt with a school on any issue before, and here we are trying to sue our school district. We had never even talked to a lawyer before. We'd never been involved in any kind of a legal matter.'"

The family lived in a small community where everybody knew everybody. Corey and his brothers had a company that had been building homes there for 15 years. One brother was a political figure. "We didn't want to get a bad reputation as the family who went and sued the local schools," Sharon says.

The AG Bell Association brought in Bruce and his partner, Jay C. Pletcher. School district officials then began responding to Sharon and Corey's complaints with literature. District officials "would give us the state handbook and say, 'Read this,' and then they'd check it off. They didn't expect us to read it or understand it, or certainly to question it."

Sharon recalls that she and Corey would attend meetings with Regan's AV therapist and a parent advocate and say, "This is not appropriate for our daughter," to which the superintendent would respond, "I have to go back and talk to someone else."

It wasn't a comfortable or easy series of negotiations. In fact, Sharon says, there were times when "it got kind of hairy. There were three-way conversations on the phone with the lawyers and that sort of thing. My husband and I would look at each other and say, 'Now what?'"

Knowing that they had the support of the AG Bell Association and two highly competent lawyers to secure the services their daughter was entitled to and needed helped Sharon and Corey. The due process procedure took 9 months, concluding when a hearing officer ruled that the cochlear implant is an assistive technology device, and therefore the school district is responsible for maintaining it in proper working order, which includes providing batteries, cords, and audiology services.

Regan never did attend public school in the district. Her parents found a private preschool they felt was more appropriate, and they also opted for private school when it came time for Regan to enter kindergarten.

"Even though we won this great case and the district was going to pay for therapy and audiology and batteries and the cords for her FM, we ended up saying that's great, that's one for the books, and hopefully this can help other families, but we had to move on," Sharon says.

Regan received a second implant between first and second grade. Now 9, she has become adept at speaking up for herself. Sharon's advocating these days consists mostly of asking her daughter's teachers to give her more challenging math problems and spelling words. In extracurricular activities, Sharon still has to remind

Regan's swimming coach to write instructions on a white board because Regan can't hear in the water, doesn't use sign language, and has to rely on written words when she isn't wearing her implants. But those issues seem minor compared to the bigger battle of taking on the local school district.

Sharon's advice for parents advocating to authorities is to become informed. Even after Bruce and Jay came on board, Sharon and Corey did not depend entirely on them. "We went back and looked at the law and learned our rights," Sharon says. "I think that's a huge part for any family—just go back to the basics, look at every law, at every rule that applies."

It's natural to begin the advocacy process with high hopes and expectations, but it's equally important to be realistic. Understanding your child's rights is critical. Listen to the people to whom you're advocating. Don't confuse compromise with weakness: compromise is a key part of the process. Your goal should be to ensure that your child receives the education, attention, or services that he needs, and to maintain a positive working relationship with the people charged with providing those services. If you find that you're constantly meeting resistance, or that a positive relationship is impossible, you may need to seek advice, either from other parents or from one of the many advocacy organizations listed in the Resources section. There *are* solutions to the problems you will encounter. Some will come more easily than others, but as with most things in life, patience, persistence, and a positive attitude will go a long way in helping you achieve your goals.

# 10

# HELPING YOUR CHILD LEARN

In the months immediately following Elizabeth's diagnosis, it seemed everything I read suggested that as a group, children with hearing loss are doomed to a bleak future. Every article seemed to cite the same studies, which had apparently all come up with nearly identical conclusions: hard-of-hearing children simply don't perform as well as their normal-hearing peers. Socially, they have problems because they often miss important cues. Academically, they lag behind because learning is language-based and much of language is picked up incidentally—that is, it's overheard. Until a child with a hearing loss is properly aided, she is at a disadvantage that will continue unless and until she's able to make up lost ground.

The studies went on to suggest that once in school, even aided and equipped with personal FM systems, children with hearing loss would continue to have problems. It wasn't just contending with background noise from classmates, overhead lights, and heating systems: when they reached fourth grade and the emphasis was on words rather than pictures, they'd be even more lost and confused.

I didn't want to believe it. Elizabeth was a bright, curious little girl with a promising future. The only thing wrong with her was that she couldn't hear as well as other children. *My kid will beat the odds*, I said to myself, all the while trying to ignore the other voice, the one that hissed, *Stop fooling yourself. It doesn't matter how smart your kid is. She's hearing impaired. Get real. Lower your expectations.*

My first glimmer of hope that there really were exceptions to the studies' gloomy predictions came from two members of a local support group for hard-of-hearing children and their families. They reminded and reassured me that all children are different, and just because a child can't hear well doesn't mean she can't learn. Gradually I began to meet parents who had hard-of-hearing teenagers who were doing well in school. I also met and, on some of the Web sites listed in the Resources section, read about hard-of-hearing adults who were successful in their studies and careers despite having grown up wearing hearing aids—and not the sophisticated models of the 21st century that are designed to be discreet and efficient and cut out as much background noise as possible. My in-laws went to a wedding reception and sat with a couple whose severely hard-of-hearing son was about to graduate from medical school, an example that made me realize that perhaps degree of hearing loss had less to do with academic success than I'd initially been led to believe.

One thing the success stories had in common was that the parents were actively involved in their children's education. They had researched forms of communication and chosen which was most appropriate for their children. They had gotten to know their children's teachers and made sure proper accommodations were in place in the classroom, whether that meant having the school supply a transliterator, translator, interpreter, or teacher of the deaf and hard of hearing or provide extra time for exams. They encouraged and supported their children at school and at home and stressed the importance of learning. Although they didn't diminish the disadvantages that come with hearing loss, neither did they allow their children to use it as an excuse not to work to their potential.

Though it would be naive to assume that every hard-of-hearing child is going to become a brain surgeon, there are things we, as parents, can and should do to ensure that our children get a proper education. Among the most important: we have to understand their hearing loss and any other disabilities they may have, be involved throughout their school career, teach them to advocate for themselves, and ensure that proper accommodations are in place so that they have the same opportunity to learn as their normal-hearing classmates.

## Hearing Loss Is *Not* a Learning Disability

Some children with hearing loss have learning disabilities. Many receive educational services from some of the same specialists who serve children with learning disabilities. But—and this is a big but

—*hearing loss is not a learning disability*, and parents should not be confused into thinking that the two automatically go hand in hand. Hearing loss is a physical condition. Not being able to hear well can certainly affect the way a child learns. That's why appropriate accommodations are essential. For families who choose to communicate using spoken language, accommodations begin with the right hearing technologies: hearing aids, cochlear implants, FM systems. Once accommodations are in place your child should be able to take full advantage of the educational system.

Children with hearing loss display the same range of intelligence as do normal-hearing children, says Christie Yoshinaga-Itano, a professor in the Department of Speech, Language and Hearing Sciences at the University of Colorado-Boulder. However, regardless of how bright hard-of-hearing children are, there are often large discrepancies between their nonverbal and verbal intelligence scores.

In people with sensory hearing loss, the cochlea doesn't work properly, either because of a malformation, or because the hair cells never formed or formed but were subsequently damaged. A child with sensorineural hearing loss will, therefore, miss out on certain sounds. Hearing aids or a cochlear implant will help, but even with the best hearing technologies, noise and distance will present problems that prevent children with hearing loss from hearing like their normal-hearing peers. Children who have frequent otitis media in addition to sensorineural hearing loss are at additional risk because, in addition to the medical implications, the otitis media adds additional conductive hearing loss. Adults experiencing late-onset hearing loss can sometimes compensate for missing words or parts of words in conversation because those neural pathways already exist: language is already fully developed and it's easier to fill in gaps, as all of us do in noisy environments where we can't hear well. Children just learning language don't have that luxury, and it is critical that they get the full range of sounds to develop those pathways.

Properly fitted hearing aids or cochlear implants allow the brain to make use of sounds that would otherwise be missed. In short, they make sounds detectable: the sounds your child needs to hear—the teacher, a friend, you—as well as the background noises, such as people chattering, dogs barking, and car horns honking, that often threaten to overwhelm the principal speaker's voice. For people with normal hearing, the brain automatically lowers background noise, allowing the listener to focus on what she wants to hear. Hearing aids and implants, for all their technological sophistication, will never work as well as a fully functioning auditory system. That means children wearing hearing aids or using a cochlear implant in a classroom, which by nature is full of background noise, will need special accommodations.

As noted earlier, in the United States those accommodations are spelled out for the school-age child in an individualized education plan (IEP). In Canada, the name of the document will vary depending on where you live, but the accommodations—FM, note-takers, transliterators or translators or interpreters, and reduced background noise—will be similar. In either country, as a parent, you are expected to work with your child's teachers to determine what accommodations will best meet your child's educational needs and be included in the plan.

Children with hearing loss even in the severe range can often function well in a school environment with assistive learning devices such as a personal FM system or a sound field FM system. They also often benefit from preferential seating close to the primary speaker and away from noise sources such as computers, heating systems, pencil sharpeners, and doors that open into a hallway. Other accommodations may include being given extra time on tests, and repeated or additional instructions. Children with the most severe hearing losses often need more accommodations. Options for these children are described in the following sections.

## Cued Speech Transliterator

The transliterator constantly converts spoken information, verbatim, to visual information using hand shapes and locations near the mouth in an effort to enhance lipreading. The transliterator, who should be beside or slightly in front of the teacher or primary source of information, provides the student with instant visual access to audible information.

## Oral Interpreter

The oral interpreter will face your child and mouth the words spoken by the teacher or other students. Oral interpreters are used by some deaf or hard-of-hearing people who don't use sign language.

## A Sign Language Interpreter or Translator

The terms *interpreter* and *translator* are often used interchangeably when describing a person who translates between oral and manual forms of communication. Because interpreter is the most commonly used term, we will use that for the purposes of this definition. However, regardless of the term used, the job is basically the same: to take an oral form of communication and represent it on the hands, either in sign language or in a sign system, and to take the form of manual communication and translate it into oral language.

If your child uses a manual form of communication, an interpreter should be by his side in school, translating what he says into the oral language being used, and what the teacher and other students say into his accepted form of manual communication. The interpreter's job is to ensure that your child has access to all that is being said, that the teacher and classmates have access to his input, and that he is able to participate in discussions.

The interpreter should be certified in the sign language or sign system used and should not change the information or apply her own interpretation to what is being said or signed. As with any profession, some interpreters are better than others. It's important to check your interpreter's credentials and references to make sure she is qualified for the job. In the United States, the Registry of Interpreters of the Deaf certifies American Sign Language (ASL) interpreters. In Canada, the certifying body for ASL is the Association of Visual Language Interpreters of Canada. The SEE Center for the Advancement of Deaf Children (http://www.seecenter.org) offers workshops and evaluations in Signing Exact English. See the Resources section in the back for more information. It's also important to check with your child and her teachers to make sure the interpreter or translator is performing her duties appropriately.

## Note Taker

In secondary schools and in the university setting it is usually possible to arrange for note takers, usually other students willing to share their notes. This can be accomplished by providing photocopies or, if the note taker is using a laptop computer, by e-mailing a copy of the notes. Using a note taker allows the student with hearing loss to focus on the teacher and supplemental visual aids.

## Real-Time Captioning

A real-time captioner uses a stenography-like machine to type the teacher's words into a computer, as the teacher is speaking. The captioning is displayed on a screen in front of the classroom, or on your child's personal computer screen, so your child can pick up information at the same time as the rest of the class.

## Video Captioning

Videos that are narrated by an unseen narrator are often difficult for hard-of-hearing students to follow. Captioning allows a student to follow the action by reading what's being said, instead of straining to listen to words that may not always be clear.

Children with hearing loss often look, act, and speak like their normal-hearing peers. For a parent having difficulty with acceptance of the hearing loss, having a child who appears to be like everyone else is a wonderful thing. But the fact remains that a child with a hearing loss has needs that are significantly different from those of his normal-hearing peers. Ultimately, it's going to be better for everyone if those differences are apparent and attended to immediately. For instance, it's not unusual for undiagnosed hard-of-hearing children to be misdiagnosed with attention deficit disorder or other behavioral problems. Some of these children may indeed have attention problems, but often the root cause of their less-than-acceptable classroom behavior is that their needs aren't being met.

That was the case with Jill's son, Ian, whose mild hearing loss wasn't diagnosed until he was 7. Before that, his teachers were convinced he had a form of attention deficit disorder described as "inattentive." That's because he wasn't hyperactive; he just didn't pay attention. After he began wearing hearing aids, but before he began using an FM system, his teacher still insisted he had behavioral problems. Her complaints were that he didn't pay attention and couldn't keep his eyes on his desk.

As it turned out, Ian's behavior was a reaction to his teacher: she paced back and forth when she spoke and often wrote on the blackboard as she talked, her back to the class. Both postures made it nearly impossible for Ian to follow what was happening. His solution was to watch his classmates for clues. But when they were reading out loud, which the teacher often had them do, he couldn't hear them. Rather than disturb the class, he doodled, which the teacher considered yet another sign of his poor attention skills.

It took Ian's parents 3 years of fighting to get the district to meet their son's needs. In addition to the FM, Ian works every day with a teacher of the deaf, and he has a number of classroom accommodations including extra time for schoolwork and on tests, one-on-one administering of any oral portions of work, and alternative test settings as needed and determined by the teacher of the deaf.

Now a senior in high school, Ian has been diagnosed with a progressive conductive hearing loss that will leave him deaf. However, he still has enough hearing to use hearing aids. "He is graduating in the top 15% of his class," his mother says proudly.

Ian's plan is to go to college and become a pediatric audiologist —not bad for a young man whose teachers once dismissed him as a problem student.

Well-behaved hard-of-hearing students are also often at a disadvantage, at least until they learn to advocate for themselves. A few years ago when I taught Hebrew school, I had a sweet, quiet student named Nicole, who preferred to doodle rather than contribute to class discussions. Yet she did well in my class, and also in public school. At the time, her mom, Pam, told me that her grades "haven't suffered yet due to her hearing impairment," but "yet" was a key to Pam's fears.

"Sometimes I feel that this has led to her teacher not attending to her needs," Pam said. "I don't think she perceives Nicole to have special needs. In the long run, this will hurt Nicole."

The year Nicole was in second grade, she had a teacher who did not consistently use either the personal FM system or the sound field system in Nicole's classroom. Pam asked repeatedly, but even when she showed up in the classroom to pick up Nicole early for an appointment, more often than not the teacher wasn't wearing the microphone. Pam spoke to the principal, but the situation didn't improve. At the end of the school year, Pam enrolled Nicole and her younger sister, who has normal hearing, in a new school where the teachers were much more supportive.

"Because of all the trouble I've had with Nicole's school, I'm not sure I'm the best one to give advice to others," Pam said. "I would say that we are the only ones who can be our child's advocate, and we have to take on that role wholeheartedly. We have to trust our instincts, encourage our child to communicate, and encourage open communication with the school and the teachers."

Open communication with your child's teachers is critical. Some parents choose to send a notebook back and forth as a way of keeping in touch with teachers and specialists. Others volunteer in the school, or schedule regular meetings. The arrangement you make will depend on your child, her teachers, and your respective schedules. Regardless of how you handle the relationship, your goal is to make sure that your child gets a solid education. That means working cooperatively with the professionals responsible for that education.

"My advice is to be the teacher's support, not adversary," says Karen, whose daughter received hearing aids at 5 months and a cochlear implant when she was 7. Now in high school, Christina is a B+ student who gets excellent support from her teachers, including an itinerant teacher, and the principal.

When Christina was in elementary and junior high school, she brought her schoolbooks home during the summer for review. Karen allowed her to invite friends over after school, as long as they did their homework first.

"It's a lot of extra work at home, but it's worth it to see her succeed," says Karen, who recommends setting aside time each day to sit down with your child for homework. "Encourage reading and make school your number one priority. It will pay off."

Children learn differently. Some hearing-impaired children excel in gym, whereas others have a lousy sense of balance. Some have excellent handwriting and thrive in art class; others have poorly developed fine motor skills. Some love to read and have no trouble sounding out words, and others will do anything to avoid cracking a book. Some love math, whereas others struggle to add single digit numbers. How your child fares in school depends on a wide range of factors, not just how well (or poorly) she hears.

## The Preschool Program: Getting on the Right Track

About a month after Elizabeth received her hearing aids, she was assigned a speech-language pathologist (SLP) at the Glenrose Rehabilitation Hospital, where her audiologist and social worker were based. As we got more involved with Elizabeth's preschool education, and as her hearing aids began to take up more of our time, sometimes requiring weekly trips to the audiology clinic, I realized how fortunate we were to live in a big city with easy access to the services we needed. I couldn't imagine how we'd cope if we lived in a remote rural area and had to drive hours to get to a clinic.

Elizabeth's new SLP was Rachel. She had a well-equipped office and classroom facilities at the Glenrose, but for her first meeting with Elizabeth, she came to our house. Her explanation: even though Elizabeth was the one with the hearing loss, we, her family, would play a role in helping her make up for the language skills she'd missed during her first 3 years. Together, we'd all work to bring her up to an age-appropriate level.

At first I feared that meant I'd have to spend hours each day going over flash cards with Elizabeth, or labeling every item in the house and conducting daily quizzes. As much as I wanted to help Elizabeth attain an age-appropriate vocabulary, I couldn't figure out where I'd find the time for that kind of intensive therapy. But although labeling certainly helps, and flash cards were truly useful, the big change in my life was that I suddenly became more aware of language. Where once I might have worked quietly or muttered under my breath as I cooked or cleaned or grocery shopped, I now made a conscious effort to talk as I went, to explain what I was doing, what we were seeing, and why.

Noah, with his normal hearing, would pick up most of his vocabulary as if by osmosis, simply by soaking up everything around him. Words like *hi*, *bye*, *kiss*, *macaroni*, *milk*, *cereal*—those words Elizabeth knew, because I'd said them to her over and over: "Here's your cereal and your milk," "Say bye to grandma," "Give Daddy a kiss." I couldn't be so sure she'd know more incidental words, like *belt buckle*, *doorknob*, *happy*, and *sad*. Those were the sorts of words Rachel began helping her with in their early sessions, the spring that Elizabeth was 3.

The following fall, Elizabeth was enrolled in the Glenrose Hospital's preschool program for children with hearing loss. There were five children in the class, all of them 3 years old or close to it. Two mornings a week, they met in a spacious but cozy classroom divided into sections for reading, playing, music, vocabulary, and snacks. First thing in the morning, Rachel inspected everyone's hearing aids and FM systems. At the same time, Brenda, the other SLP in the program, began one-on-one speech therapy sessions in a smaller room down the hall. The children used their free time to play, look at books, or sit on the lap of a parent, grandparent, or aide and listen to a story.

Once class was in session, the five children sat side by side in a row of chairs while Rachel took attendance. When their names were called, they had to respond. It was good training for elementary school, but its intended purpose was to train the children to listen for their name and respond appropriately. Late-diagnosed children, so accustomed to not hearing, often tune out without even thinking about it. They need to be taught how to listen, something that comes naturally to normal-hearing children (though parents might often think otherwise).

After attendance, the children continued sitting while Rachel read them a story or reviewed new words, always using pictures to reinforce the vocabulary. Sometimes the three boys in the class moved around and bothered each other, but within a few months, fidgeting happened rarely, if at all. By and large, the five children, some of whom had yet to reach their 3rd birthday, were unwaveringly attentive.

Just how remarkable this was became clear to me a year later, when Elizabeth was in kindergarten. Because her birthday was close to the cutoff date, she was at least a half year younger than some of her classmates. And yet most of them seemed much less able to sit still and cooperate than her hard-of-hearing classmates had been.

"They knew they had to listen," Brenda explained to me when I asked her about it a few years later. Few children are in such structured preschool programs that put so much emphasis on listening. "We're expecting active participation in listening, and a response. In a playschool, you don't necessarily get an opportunity to answer a question—you're given that opportunity, but not everybody gets picked. In our program, everybody got picked. When our kids get to elementary school, the teachers love them, because they know how to sit and pay attention and focus."

After vocabulary, the children did a craft, something that reinforced whatever concept they were learning. One of Elizabeth's favorites was the first craft she did, a picture of a house in which she had to paste the appropriate furniture in each room: the stove and fridge in the kitchen, the toilet and sink and tub in the bathroom, the bed and desk and dresser in the bedroom. It sounds so obvious, and to children who hear and pick up language incidentally, it is. Children who are hard of hearing need these things pointed out, and reinforced over and over, until it becomes second nature to them.

The preschool program also included physical education, music, and drama. Rachel and Brenda videotaped the kids' performances in *We're Going on a Bear Hunt, The Three Little Pigs,* and *The Very Hungry Caterpillar,* so they could have permanent records of their acting debuts.

When, at the end of the preschool year, Dave and I were informed that Elizabeth had tested at or above her age level in speech and language and therefore didn't need to come back to the program the following year, I cried. Elizabeth had gotten a first-rate education in the preschool program, and I doubted she'd ever again be in a situation with such a favorable teacher-to-student ratio—five children, a teacher, an aide, an SLP, and at least one parent and grandparent at every session to help out.

"This is a good thing," Rachel and Brenda insisted, as they handed me a box of tissues. "She's ready to be mainstreamed."

The question for Dave and me was, mainstreamed in what? It was nearly the end of June. The other preschool programs in the city were closed for the summer, so it was too late to even observe them. It was also too late to get Elizabeth into a private kindergarten, as admissions had closed months earlier.

Our neighborhood playschool, where Elizabeth had gone one day a week in addition to the Glenrose program, was strictly for play. The focus was on fun, crafts, and games. After a year where Elizabeth had thrived in a highly structured environment, Dave and I worried that a year of fun and games would be a step backward, not to mention less than stimulating for her.

I spent a lot of time that summer seeking the opinions of everyone we could think of, including a friend who is a child psychiatrist and had been saying since May that Elizabeth was ready for kindergarten. She wouldn't turn 5 until mid-January, but our school district's cutoff date is March 1, so technically her age wasn't a problem. And Dave and I, whose birthdays are in December and November, had both started school early and managed to do well. I worried that she might not be able to keep up, but I was more concerned that she'd be bored and backslide in playschool. I felt as if we had no choice but to enroll her in kindergarten.

A week before Labor Day, I went to our neighborhood school to register her. The receptionist handed me a form, and I began to fill it out.

"Elizabeth is hearing impaired," I explained to the principal. "She has a personal FM system. I can come and show the teacher how to use it."

That's when the administrative assistant spoke up. "My daughter is hearing impaired," she said, smiling warmly at me. "She has an FM, too."

I felt my eyes well up with tears. The administrative assistant had a daughter who wore hearing aids? In such a small school, there would be someone who would understand not only how to help Elizabeth, but what I was going through as well? I couldn't believe my good fortune. And it got better: one of the two teachers who job-shared in the kindergarten/grade one classroom had taught at the provincial School for the Deaf, and had also taught in a mainstream school with hard-of-hearing children.

In the years since Elizabeth started school, the administrative assistant, Jan, has become a friend, a shoulder to lean on, and the person Elizabeth went to for help with equipment checks and battery changes. Because Jan's daughter, Melissa, is 10 years older than Elizabeth, Jan had been down the road on which I was just starting: she was the person who let me know when it was time to start encouraging Elizabeth to take responsibility for battery changes, and she warned me of what I could expect when Elizabeth reached high school and would protest about using her FM. In fact, Elizabeth began protesting about the FM in fifth grade, but I wasn't as surprised as I would have been had nobody warned me.

Our fears that Elizabeth wasn't academically ready for school were unfounded. Her teachers made that clear to us throughout kindergarten, and as the years have gone by, it's obvious they're right. Elizabeth is an A student, responsible and conscientious. She enjoys her schoolwork and takes pride in it. She likes art, music, and reading, but her favorite subjects seem to change: one week she likes language arts and writing stories, the next week she likes math.

That's not to say she hasn't had any problems. Her spelling is inconsistent, and in elementary school she didn't always follow directions properly, but no one, from her teachers to the district's educational consultant for the deaf and hard of hearing, has been able to say for sure whether either issue is a function of her age and development or her hearing loss. I'm tempted to go more with the former, and not just because her teachers have assured us that such problems are common among primary school students. Halfway through second grade, the educational consultant for the deaf and hard of hearing came to school to observe Elizabeth and test her. On the Kaufman Test of Educational Achievement, she tested above her age level in spelling and math computation.

## Danny: Following the Academic Path Set by His Hearing Brother

Danny was born with what's known as a Mondini malformation: he has no cochlea in his right ear and a partial formation in his left. He was diagnosed as profoundly deaf when he was about a year old. Five months before his 2nd birthday, he received a cochlear implant. Until then, he had been largely silent. "The only time we heard his voice was when he laughed or cried," says his mother, Jennifer, an occupational therapist.

Once Danny received his implant, a teacher from the Boys Town National Research Hospital Early Education Program came to the family's house weekly to work with Danny and the family. Her goal was to alert Danny to sound and help him and his family with his communication and language skills.

Six months after he was implanted. Danny was enrolled in a toddler program at Boys Town, where the emphasis was on total communication. Eventually his parents signed him up for two other, separate, programs. At the Omaha Hearing School, which he attended part-time for 3 years, he focused on auditory training. At the Jewish Community Center in Omaha, which he attended part-time for 2 years, he received an introduction to the Jewish education that is part of his family heritage.

By the time Danny entered kindergarten shortly before his 6th birthday, he'd had 3 years of preschool in three different programs. He'd been reading for almost 2 years, and was eager to learn more. To further ease his transition into the public school system, the district put together a sign language class for his kindergarten classmates. Fifteen students showed up for the class, which took place during the summer. Danny and his mother helped teach. The class wasn't intended to make the students proficient. Rather, it was an introduction designed to provide a comfort level so the youngsters would understand the basics of sign language and not spend class time trying to figure out who Danny's interpreter was and what she was doing. It also had the perhaps unexpected benefit of showing Danny's classmates that even though he didn't hear well, he had something to offer.

That he was smart was never in question. He surprised even his family when, at 4, he began to read to his mother. She hadn't taught him. In fact, she always worried he'd have trouble with reading because phonetics is sound-based. But because reading is important to the family, she read to him constantly, finger-spelling words for which there were no signs in Signing Exact English. One day she finger spelled *b-u-s*, and Danny, unprompted, said, "bus."

Soon the family began holding finger-spelling contests, where Danny competed with his brother, who is 2½ years older, and his dad. "He was just great," Jennifer says. "I would finger spell, say, *plumber*, and he would come back and say 'plumb-ber'. Having never heard the word, he didn't know not to pronounce the *b*."

Entering kindergarten, Danny tested above average in every subject except for math, where his scores were average. In first grade, he began having trouble with math. Jennifer asked the teacher to send home more worksheets, and she began looking for opportunities to work math into what they were doing at home. For example, using play money, Jennifer and Danny would play "grocery store." Danny would have to count out dollars needed to "buy" something or he would have to count back change. Jennifer would quiz Danny on simple things such as how many items they had if they had three packages with eight items in each.

Jennifer spoke with the district's consultant for the deaf and hard of hearing about Danny's difficulty in math, but it wasn't clear whether the problems stemmed from his hearing loss or whether he'd have trouble even if his hearing were normal. The consultant suggested that some of the information he needed may have been getting lost in translation, and that because he is such a visual learner, the concepts were more difficult when they were merely explained. Danny does much better if he can see the problem—laying out coins that are to be added up, for example.

When Danny was in second grade, his parents enrolled him a math program run by Kumon, a private tutoring company. By fifth grade he excelled at the subject and had begun participating in a challenge math program at his school. Reading and writing continued to be difficult, however. "He reads constantly, and enjoys it," Jennifer says, "but he does not score well on reading tests—at least not as well as I think he should be able to. As for writing, he has a ton of creative ideas, but getting them onto paper is difficult." Danny gets taken out of class every week for sessions with a speech-language therapist and a counselor for the deaf.

Jennifer and her husband, John, had worried even before Danny was ready for kindergarten about the effects of making the transition from small, specialized programs with five children to a large public school class with more than 20. Their local school district had a large population of deaf and hard-of-hearing children, but its program was primarily sign-based, and Danny's parents wanted him to focus on oral skills. They ruled out a school where he would have to share an interpreter with several other students, and finally decided to send him to the neighborhood school. "The services were good, and he could go to school with his brother and kids in the neighborhood," Jennifer says.

At the time, Danny was the only deaf child so he had his own interpreter. Eventually another deaf child enrolled at the school. The school hired an additional interpreter, so both he and Danny have their own.

"The choice has turned out to be a good one for Danny," Jennifer says. "It is basically an oral setting with regular hearing peers and the interpreter for backup when Danny has a hard time understanding his peers or the teacher. In this setting Danny only speaks, which is his choice of communication style."

Danny's interpreter signs to him so he'll know what's being said, but he speaks to her, his teachers, and classmates. "Basically we sign to him and he talks to us," his mother says. "He's still pretty good at lip reading and does pretty well at school communicating with classmates and friends."

In social situations, "the interpreter is there to help if needed," says Jennifer, but she has done her best to prevent the interpreter from becoming "Danny's little buddy," by his side at all times for social interactions. "I was afraid he'd end up interacting with the interpreter instead of with the kids," she says. So far that has not happened.

Still, social life has been challenging, particularly at the start of the school year, when it takes a while for Danny to work out who he'll interact with at recess. He doesn't like sports, so he doesn't join in impromptu ball games, nor does he like group activities. Now in fifth grade, he has been with the same classmates for 6 years. "They know and like him, and respect him," Jennifer says, but in addition to not joining in games at the playground, he chooses not to participate in activities such as Scouts and districtwide reading competitions that would provide more opportunities to develop relationships. "I don't know if this is due to his being deaf, or just his personality," Jennifer says. "I do know that he has difficulty with group interactions, following conversations. He prefers one-on-one interactions."

Not long after his 6th birthday, Danny asked to take Suzuki piano lessons. His brother had been taking lessons for 4 years. Jennifer had reservations, but did not want to treat Danny differently because of his deafness. "I don't want his life to be different because of my preconceived notions that he can't do something," she said at the time. "If it's just a frustration and he isn't getting anywhere, we won't continue."

Five years later, Danny is still enjoying lessons. He learns by reading music, tapping out the rhythm, and practicing small parts of a song at a time. "I know if he could hear the music it would be much easier for him, but with enough repetition and his implant, he does become familiar with what a song is supposed to sound like," Jennifer says. "Sometimes his hands are misplaced by one note and he has no idea how awful that can sound! However, he is doing very well, and even participated in a five-piano concert, playing a duet with nine other boys at the same time."

By age 11, Danny was beginning to prepare for his Bar Mitzvah, a Jewish coming-of-age ceremony that takes place when a boy turns 13. He was learning to read Hebrew and chant prayers. "This is difficult, as most kids learn by listening to the words and melodies," Jennifer says. "However, with lots of practice and repetition, I know he will be able to do this, too."

## Julie: Facing a Variety of Challenges

Julie's parents took her to an audiologist for her first hearing test when she was 3, but it wasn't until she was 4 that she received an accurate diagnosis: a moderate-to-profound sensorineural loss in her right ear and a severe-to-profound mixed loss in her left. It took a month for the audiologist to fit her with appropriate hearing aids.

In the meantime, her mother, Elyse, who knew nothing about hearing loss or the educational needs of children, recalls, "I was scared out of my mind. The experts told me she had too much hearing to go to a deaf school, and even if she went to a deaf school, she'd come out with a fourth-grade reading level."

After much research, Elyse and her husband, Larry, decided to send Julie to their local public school. The district provided Julie with an itinerant teacher for the deaf, who spent 3 hours a week in the classroom with her, or took her out of class to work with her privately. Julie's IEP says the school must provide captioning for videos, extra time for tests, and preferential seating, and that directions must be reread or simplified as needed. Early in Julie's school years, Elyse lobbied the district to buy a wireless FM instead of the less expensive and less effective older version it would have preferred to purchase.

Elyse also made a point of advanced planning: at the end of each academic year, she knew who Julie's teacher would be for the following year, and what friends would be in her class. But on the first day of second grade, the principal informed Elyse that Julie would be in a different class. The problem: the teacher whose class she was supposed to be in refused to wear the FM microphone. A cancer survivor, the teacher had gone through chemotherapy the year before and was afraid the microphone would emit radiation.

It was an irrational fear—the FM emits nothing harmful—but it nonetheless resulted in upheaval at the beginning of Julie's school year. Then, in fifth grade, Julie failed math in the first marking period. Elyse believes it's because she didn't feel prepared and wasn't up to the challenge, coming off a year with a teacher who had spoken in a monotone that she'd found hard to understand.

After the first report cards went home, Julie worked hard with her itinerant teacher and stayed after school 2 days a week for a small class with other students who needed extra help. By the end of the year, she earned a B. By eighth grade, she was an A student who scored in the superior range in districtwide language arts exams. Her mother was grateful for and pleased with her daughter's academic success.

Socially, school was more challenging. In one-on-one situations, Julie did well, but in large groups she had trouble hearing and keeping up. Strong-willed and outgoing, she preferred to dominate a conversation, perhaps, Elyse says, "because it's the only way you can hear what's going on." It wasn't an entirely successful method. Julie had a couple of friends, "a teeny little clique," her mother said.

The summer before Julie entered eighth grade, her parents arranged for her to have a cochlear implant in her left ear. She had become a candidate when the hearing in her better ear, her right, deteriorated during elementary school. Julie continues to use a hearing aid in her right ear.

The implant did wonders for Julie's hearing and for her social life. Once upon a time, that would have made Elyse happy, but in high school it proved to be a disaster. In mid-ninth grade, Julie became a social butterfly. As she grew more used to the implant and began hearing better, her confidence improved and her group of friends grew. Her new friends took precedence over school. Her grades took a nose-dive. Elyse thinks she was making up for lost time, all the years when she didn't have many friends and spent most of her time doing homework.

Elyse tried, unsuccessfully, to convince her daughter to pay more attention to academics. "I used the term 'falling on deaf ears.' To her, I was another old person lecturing her."

By Julie's senior year in high school, her grades were so bad that there was a chance she wouldn't be able to graduate. Meanwhile, schoolmates who had worked hard were going off to college and being rewarded for doing well. Some even got cars. That proved to be the wake-up call Julie needed.

Midway through her last year in high school, Julie was back on track. However, she still refused to use her FM or the captioning services that the district was willing to provide. Elyse wouldn't push her to use them. "I can't hold a gun to her head and insist that she does it," she says. "At home she uses captioning all the time, but in front of her friends she's embarrassed."

Perhaps if Elyse were convinced that Julie's poor performance had to do with not taking advantage of the services to which she is entitled, she might have reacted differently. But that's not the case. "It had nothing to do with it," she says. "It was a typical teenage rebellion."

And it appears to be over. "She was an A and B student, a fantastic student, and she is climbing back up, thank God," Elyse says. "I think maturity and seeing some other friends going away and doing better and getting all the things you get when you're responsible and mature made a difference. She's going to classes and doing her homework. That's going in the right direction."

# Melissa: School Was a Constant Struggle, but Mom Learned an Important Lesson: Ask Questions until You Get Answers

Melissa was diagnosed with a mild-to-moderate loss when she was about 2½, after a day care worker noticed she didn't seem to be able to hear when someone called her from across the room. Her mother, my friend Jan, who was by then separated from Melissa's dad, got her the help she needed right away, "but it was a roller coaster for a very long time," she recalls.

"You'd have these highs—'Melissa is doing so well. She's got her speech patterns fixed, she's saying everything the way she's supposed to say it, she's not going to have any problems with her speech.' And then it would be, 'But she has trouble with concepts, she has trouble with word recognition, she has trouble with letter recognition.' So it went back and forth between 'She's doing great,' 'Oh, she's not doing great'; I was constantly feeling, 'Where am I? What do I do now?'"

Like Elizabeth, Melissa went to the Glenrose Rehabilitation Hospital in Edmonton for hearing tests and speech therapy. The professionals spoke in diagnostic terms Jan often found difficult to decipher, and they sent her reports predicting future problems she could expect Melissa to encounter. Because Jan had no experience with the education system, she found it hard to relate to the predictions.

By the time Melissa reached first grade, the problems were beginning. She couldn't sound out words. Even with her hearing aids, certain sounds didn't register, making phonetic reading difficult.

"You could say yes, that's typical of a hearing-impaired child," Jan says, "but you can have the kid sitting next to her who's not hearing impaired who has the same reading problems. So you don't really know why it's happening."

Melissa learned to read, but unlike her mother, who calls herself "a readaholic," she never learned to love it. Jan believes that had a lasting effect on her academic achievement. "You know that kids with hearing loss are going to have trouble with vocabulary—they're only going to want to learn the words that can help them get their point across in the fastest and simplest way. They're not going to want to learn 12 words for silly."

At Melissa's elementary school, all sorts of promises were made, from the guarantee of extra help in language arts to the promises of an individualized program plan, "but it never came to pass," Jan says.

Not only did school officials renege on their promises, she says, judging from the comments on Melissa's progress reports— "'Melissa needs to study more' and 'Melissa needs to put more effort into preparing for exams'—they seemed to have overlooked the underlying reasons for her learning problem."

By the time Melissa was in sixth grade, her FM was so old Jan was told it wasn't worth repairing. The school refused to buy a new system, but it did agree to purchase a second-hand one on the condition that Jan reimburse them before Melissa moved on to junior high school. She agreed only because she wanted to make sure Melissa would get an FM as quickly as possible.

Then she called the district's audiology consultant, who informed her that the school was responsible for purchasing equipment required for instructional use and that it could not refuse or "blackmail" parents into paying for it. Jan told the elementary school principal she wouldn't reimburse the school. "I told them if they wanted to pursue it, they could talk to the audiology consultant," she recalls. "I never heard another word about it."

In seventh grade, Melissa used an FM owned by the junior high school. She also had time with an aide every day. But the following year the aide position was eliminated due to budget cuts, and the FM broke and was going to take weeks to repair. There is a provincial agency that helps parents purchase FM systems for their children, but only if the systems will be used outside of school. So Jan sent the agency a proposal.

"I had to come up with situations where she would use it outside of school, even though I knew those situations weren't likely," Jan says. "But Melissa needed the FM, and we couldn't afford to pay for it ourselves." The proposal was accepted, and Melissa got a new FM.

However, her academic problems persisted. Though she scored well on class work, she consistently failed tests because she didn't understand the questions. Jan was convinced there were holes in Melissa's vocabulary. The principal offered to have someone read the exam questions to Melissa, but what Jan wanted was to have the questions rephrased. She was repeatedly told it could not be done.

Jan, who was working for the school board's Department of Continuing Education, was beginning to feel like a pest. She was pushing the principal to have Melissa tested by school board professionals to pinpoint specific areas of need before she moved on to high school, but he wasn't moving very quickly. When she finally did get a positive response, it was because the principal was out of town and his e-mail was automatically forwarded to one of the counselors, who e-mailed back promptly and said, "No problem. I'll set that up right away."

"So that's a really important lesson," Jan says. "If you keep banging on the door and you're not getting in, try a different door. It turned out you don't talk to the principals of the schools. Once you get to junior high, you talk to the counselors. And where I made my mistake in the first 2 years of junior high school was I kept talking to the principal. He'd sit there and nod and he wouldn't do anything. He never said, 'Go talk to the counselor' and he never passed my requests on to the counselor."

Jan's next eye-opening experience came before Melissa started high school. She received a call from a high school counselor recommending Melissa enter a program for students who had been in a junior high program for students with learning disabilities.

"I said, 'She's not coming out of a program for students with learning disabilities,' and the counselor said, 'Yes, she is,' and I said, 'She's not learning disabled, she's hearing impaired,' and the counselor said, 'What? She's not coded as hearing impaired.'"

"That's how I learned she wasn't coded properly," Jan says. "You, as a parent, have no way of knowing how your child is coded unless you check. And you have to check."

When Melissa was finally tested in ninth grade, Jan learned she had a long-term memory retention deficit. To accommodate for that, in high school Melissa focused on only two core subjects at a time, so the material was compacted into a shorter time frame. When final exam time rolled around, instead of having to remember material from September to June, she had to remember only from September to December, and then from January to June.

"High school was definitely the best experience in terms of our relationship with teachers," Jan says. "At this point, they could see she was a hard-working, intelligent girl who had some roadblocks to comprehension."

She was also a dedicated athlete, winning Canadian championships in five-pin bowling both as a team member and an individual. She graduated from high school in 2003, a solid C student. The following fall, she started a job in the purchasing department of an office supply company, doing data entry. Two years later, she was accepted into a technical college to study graphic design. She's now a certified graphic designer for a chain of sporting goods stores.

The years of doing poorly in school brought Jan and Melissa closer, especially the 3 years in junior high when Melissa often came home saying, "I'm stupid. I'm never going to have a good life. I can't pass anything and I can't learn anything."

"Those were the years we really bonded, because we stuck together," Jan says. Adding to Melissa's academic problems was that some of the girls she'd been friends with were becoming "clique-y" in the way that junior high school girls often do. Melissa still had some friends, but she was already feeling sensitive, and the rejection didn't help.

"I felt awful, but I wasn't going to let her sink into that 'Oh, feel sorry for me' stuff, either," Jan says. "I said, look, there are a lot of people in this world who are not academically proficient and if you don't know what that means you can look it up. But you don't have to be a university graduate to have a good life. There's lots of people out there who never even went to school that have a good life. You'll have the life that you make for yourself, and if that's in school or that's digging ditches or whatever, you'll be happy."

As for Jan, she wishes she'd been better prepared. She's generous and warm and helpful by nature, but I'm convinced part of what's led her to reach out to me and Elizabeth is that she doesn't want others to go blindly down the same path she had to carve out for herself and Melissa.

More than once she's told me, "Being aware of what could possibly be ahead of you puts you light years ahead of where I was. I had no idea Melissa was going to have problems of this magnitude. I didn't even know where to turn to deal with it. Now that I've been on both sides, as a parent and working in a school, I'd say you have to keep pushing."

# 11

# ADVICE FROM THE TRENCHES

One of the reasons I set out to write this book was to find answers to the questions that had stumped me when Elizabeth was first diagnosed. But it eventually became apparent that understanding how her inner ear worked and the difference between digital and analog hearing aids wasn't enough. What I really wanted to know was: How is the hearing loss going to affect her over the course of her life? Will she be happy? Will she be productive? Will she have good friends? What can I do to make sure everything turns out okay for her?

For those questions, of course, there are no answers. Nobody has them, even when hearing loss isn't involved. So, I decided, if I couldn't predict Elizabeth's future, I'd talk to people who grew up wearing hearing aids. I'd ask what their parents had done to help or hinder them, and what they wished the hearing people in their lives had understood about hearing loss. Our children will no doubt have different lives from the people profiled here, but in the absence of a crystal ball, their stories provide helpful insights.

## Paige

On a Friday afternoon in late November, Paige sits at her desk, surrounded by scientific articles she needs to read before writing her latest grant proposal. An assistant professor in the Department of Medicine at the University of Alberta, Paige is a principal investigator in a large research group studying chronic obstructive pulmonary disease and asthma. Her specialty: determining how white blood cells called *neutrophils* and *eosinophils* contribute to these and other lung diseases.

Her office is a hub of activity. E-mails flash on the computer monitor, which is within easy eyeshot of a framed photo of her husband and their 9-year-old daughter. When the phone rings, it's her husband, calling to let her know they've been invited to a friend's for Christmas dinner. Researchers knock on the door periodically, eager to share news of their latest finds.

"I'm getting to the stage where people are starting to sit up and notice what I'm doing, and it's just so sweet," she says. "I never expected to go this far with hearing loss."

Paige has a profound sensorineural loss in her left ear and a severe loss in her right. That she has a career she loves and a solid marriage and family life are a testament to her innate intelligence, self-described aggressive personality, and a mother who consistently bolstered her self-esteem, giving her confidence so that even when classmates ignored her and made her school years a misery, she knew she had something going for her.

"The thing my mother did was she kept on telling me that I was very bright and very clever," Paige says. "I believed it, and I think that helped."

For every Paige, a social outcast who never had a close friend until she was 12 but who excelled in school, loved books, and read herself to sleep every night, there's a Toby. A well-liked bundle of energy, Toby almost failed fifth grade and spent the next 3 years in special ed classes. Rather than feeling sorry for himself, he took advantage of the smaller classes and caring teachers. Given a chance to phase back into "the regular mainstream" in high school, which he says "was kind of like getting called up to the majors," he opted to stay in special ed for math and English.

On the surface, Toby and Paige appear to have nothing in common except hearing loss: she's a preppy-looking academic with a wall full of advanced degrees, happily married and raising a child. He's a 28-year-old television cameraman barely out of his baggy-pants-and-dyed-hair skateboarding phase, sharing an apartment with two other young men in downtown Toronto.

Yet when I asked both of them, in separate interviews, what advice they'd give parents of newly diagnosed hearing impaired children, they told me the same thing: "It's not the end of the world."

"It's not something I'd change about myself, really," Toby says. "I don't mind it. It's just who I am. If I'm in loud places, it's hard for me to hear, but it's normal for me. People ask, 'How do you get by? How do you hear?' It's like people who don't see quite as well. You kind of get used to it and move on."

Says Paige, "Those two words, hearing impaired, are so tiny, so small, compared to what the mind of a child can do. There is a sense, of course, that the social interaction is missing for those kids, but remember, as they go along in life, the people who really care are the ones who are going to be their friends. If they're born into a family that really cares about them, and shows their appreciation and is very patient with them and enjoys their company and their insight and their input into things, then I think it's very much more likely that they can go ahead."

Toby was diagnosed with hearing loss just before his 2nd birthday. His mother, Vicki, took him to the audiologist and to speech therapy. At home she labeled everything from cups to doors to help him expand his miniscule vocabulary.

"I owe so much to my mom," he says. "Only about 5 or 6 years ago did I really realize how hard she worked, how dedicated she was. It does pay off in the end."

But that doesn't mean those early years are going to be easy. For Paige, who was born in 1962, they were pretty much a nightmare. Although she was apparently born with normal hearing, by the time she was a year old, her vocabulary had stopped developing. Her parents were separated by then, and her mother bore the responsibility for getting a diagnosis.

The first doctor they visited concluded Paige was either mentally retarded or autistic. She managed to fool nearly every doctor who tested her, either by lipreading or picking up clues from her mother, on whose lap she sat for every hearing test. It was only when a specialist sent her mother out of the sound booth and covered his mouth during the test that Paige was given an accurate diagnosis. By then she was nearly 8, and she'd been wearing hearing aids for almost 5 years, although they were probably not appropriately fitted. They made everything louder, which she found overwhelming. She hated them. On more than one occasion she pulled them out of her ears and hurled them across a room. Once she bit into them so hard she left teeth marks in the plastic casing.

Her relationships with peers weren't much better. In day care she stole vitamins out of the other kids' lunches, and in grade school she was one rung above the least popular kid in class. In middle school, girls would walk away when they saw her coming. Once she went to someone's house to play, and the girl kept her waiting on the porch for a half hour, finally emerging to announce, "I've got a lot of fish bones stuck in my throat and I just don't feel very good, so I don't want to play right now."

It wasn't until she was 12 and her family moved to New Zealand that Paige finally began making friends. To this day, she thinks it had more to do with the accepting nature of the kids in her adopted country than with any change in her personality.

"They didn't have a problem with eccentricity or odd speech patterns or odd anything," she says. "They thought I had a strong American accent while I was there, and I was just the American kid and that was kind of interesting for them. It was a novelty."

Paige was born in Dallas and by the time she moved to New Zealand she'd also lived in Pasadena,CA; Santa Fe, NM; and Philadelphia. She never received special services in school because of her hearing loss. There were no FM systems, no itinerant teachers of the deaf and hard of hearing to provide one-on-one tutorials. Often she had trouble following what was being said and where discussions were going. She relied strongly on visual cues and grew to appreciate the loud, clear, and slow speech patterns of her teachers, particularly the ones in the United States.

The teachers, too, recognized her ability. Halfway through kindergarten her teacher moved her into first grade, sensing she was bored and would benefit from learning to read. Paige learned within 2 weeks, and she loved it.

"I would read until I fell asleep every night, because this was where my information flow was," she says. "The rest of the day, it was kind of patchy, and reading was nice and continuous. It's logical. There are no missing bits, all the words are there. And you can control it."

Her weaknesses were comprehension, understanding new concepts, and retaining information. Math was a consistent problem: she needed help with addition, and one summer she forgot how to do long division. To this day she considers herself a slow learner, and she's convinced her hearing loss has something to do with that.

"It's almost like a part of your brain really needs the auditory information to come in to make it work," she says. "When you don't get speech coming in, somehow your ability to process the information through speech is missing. You can read and understand information very well, though, and that's a very good compensatory mechanism. If I were a parent of a hard-of-hearing child, I would spend a lot of time getting my child really quickly up to speed on reading. I'd throw books at her right and left."

Paige's family returned to New Mexico when she was 15. At the time, she was excited, looking forward to returning home. "By this point I'd forgotten what it was like," she says. "We went back, and within 1 week I regretted it. I was in my junior year of high school, and it was just awful. No one wanted to play with me again, and this was a different group of people; the ones who were in class with me before had all gone off to different schools."

When the school year ended, Paige struck a deal with the guidance counselor to finish her credits at a local college. Eventually she moved back to New Zealand, where she graduated from Victoria University and entered the PhD program at the Wellington School of Medicine at the University of Otago. Neither university had an office of students with disabilities, so Paige came up with her own system for success.

"I copied people's notes because I couldn't hear the lecturer and write notes at the same time," she says. "I befriended students in my most charming manner possible, and they were very nice. I never got a 'no.' They were all really helpful."

As a child, Paige avoided telling people she had a hearing loss. Her husband, an engineer she met and married during graduate school, has encouraged her to be more open about it.

"He says people treat me like an idiot otherwise," she admits. But what really helped her overcome her sense of shame about her loss was meeting a highly respected European scientist who is going blind.

"When he gives presentations, he has to say, 'Please tell me if the slide is upside down, because I can't tell.' When I told people this story, they thought it was a joke, but it's not. It was like he was giving people a chance to understand his disability. He was letting them into his world, in a sense. When I sat down with him, I said, 'I was amazed at how you could say that without feeling humiliated in front of all those people,' and he said, 'Oh no, you should use it, because not only do they get less confused at why things aren't working the way they think they should, you're helping them to become more patient and understanding. So we become the teachers of other people.'"

Down-to-earth and realistic, Paige isn't the sort to put a cheerful spin on something just to make it easier to accept. So when she offers her take on the positive aspects of hearing loss, it's hard not to take them seriously. For instance, she says, she experiences a wonderful sense of peace and calm when she removes her hearing aids before going to sleep. And during the waking hours, there are also benefits.

"It opens doors in ways you might not have imagined," she says. "For example, if I walk into a group of people and start talking to a few of them and some of them talk back to me and they're not clear, and I say, 'Listen, I have a hearing loss. I can't understand what you're saying, it's very crowded, and I need you to slow down, face me, and articulate your words,' and they go 'oohghhsoxlb' and walk off, I say to myself, 'There you are. You've just done self-selection. You are not a patient and considerate and compassionate human being.' I wind up going with the patient, compassionate, kind types, because they're the ones that actually face me and speak clearly. I end up gravitating toward the really nice people."

That lesson won't be so obvious to a child at a small school where the pool of potential friends is limited. "As you get older and start working, you can move yourself in directions where the people are better at opening up and being kind to you," Paige says. "What you find as a hearing-impaired person is that gradually, gradually, gradually, you are with a group of people who are wonderful, because they're the people who are making the effort to reach out and communicate."

## Toby

If you're convinced that the biggest disadvantage to wearing hearing aids is the stigma, you've probably never worn hearing aids. So before you risk prejudicing your hard-of-hearing child with unfounded worries, consider what Toby—who has worn hearing aids for 26 of his 28 years—has to say:

"Sweat is the biggest disadvantage of having hearing aids. Water-resistant aids would be a dream. Waterproof aids would be even better."

Mind you, Toby is an avid athlete who grew up playing just about every sport imaginable and continues to play hockey year-round, but sweat is a universal problem, so common that audiology clinics generally carry at least one device to protect equipment from moisture. But Toby has yet to find the ideal product, so when he plays hockey, he wears only one aid. If he misses out on rink chatter, that's fine with him.

"Half the time you don't even want to hear what people are saying," he says. "It doesn't bother me that much."

Not that Toby is a recluse. In fact, he's an outgoing young man who shares a house with two other people and likes going out with his buddies. If he misses out on conversations, he'll ask the speaker to repeat what he's said, up to 10 times if necessary, though generally he settles for three.

"My lipreading isn't that good," he says. "I'm always running into people who mumble or don't move their lips correctly. I live in Toronto, and accents are a tricky business, too. Usually what I do is stick my ear in the speaker's mouth and they usually yell and I usually hear it. It can be bad, but I'm not a big fan of crowded places anyway. I don't go out to loud bars. If anything, the one disadvantage when I go out is that it's hard to hear, but I just go with it, and that's about it. You can't really change much."

It's become something of a cliché to say that life works best if you accept what you can't change and change what you can, but that philosophy seems to have worked for Toby. Consider his early academic career: he was a poor student, though he's reluctant to blame that on his hearing loss. "My brother was the same way, so maybe it was genetic," he reasons.

Whatever the cause, Toby was a hyperactive boy who would rather have been playing hockey or soccer or riding his bike than sitting quietly at a desk in a classroom. "In grade five I had a really tough year. I nearly got put back, so I did special ed in grade six, seven, and eight, and it made all the difference for me."

The special ed classes were small, and Toby benefited from the extra attention. Rather than dwelling on the negative and feeling badly about being put in special ed, he focused on learning as much as he could.

"All the special ed teachers were so cool. They were patient and easygoing. That made you want to go to school and go to class and learn more," he says. "By grade seven I was doing all right, and by the time I got to high school my grades went up. I think I started trying harder. I think the motivation was realizing that this was when school really counted."

The school board provided Toby with an FM system, which he says he began "getting fed up with" halfway through elementary school. That was understandable: the FM of the era consisted of a box attached to the body with four straps that Toby likens to "a strap-on-bomb-type device." In fifth grade he received a more modern model with boots that attached to his hearing aids, but by high school he was ready to abandon the system altogether.

"I'd always be sitting at the front, and it became more of a hassle to put it away every night and to get it from every teacher at the end of the class," he says. In college, he opted to forego the FM in favor of sitting in the front of the room.

"I have a moderate-to-severe hearing loss but I can still hear people pretty good and if there's no yapping in the class, I can hear fine," he says. "In real life I'm not going to have an FM. I don't want one and I don't need one, and I'm not going to get one unless I fork over a ton of money."

About a half dozen kids at Toby's elementary school wore hearing aids, and when he started kindergarten he was just one of the younger kids with a hearing loss.

"It was kind of accepted throughout the school," he says. "I was never picked on, and by grade seven or eight it was a normal thing. By high school, everyone grows up, they figure out what hearing aids are, and that's that. I used it to my advantage, if anything, when I was a kid."

The FM system made Toby more attractive to his classmates. By third grade they'd figured out that if they put their ears up to his, they could hear everything the teacher said when she left the room if she forgot to turn off the microphone, which she generally did.

At a hockey game when he was 16, he used his hearing loss to help his team. "I was mad and I shot the puck after the whistle, and the ref gave me a penalty," he recalls. "I heard my coach yell, 'He can't hear, he can't hear, he wears hearing aids,' and I thought, 'I have to use this to my advantage.' The ref said, 'Can you hear?' and

I said, 'No.' Later my coach told me he knew I'd heard the whistle, but he figured it was worth a try. That was the only time I got away with it."

It wasn't, however, the only time someone asked him if he couldn't hear. One summer when he was in his late teens he worked at a gas station. During rush hour on a busy afternoon when the streets were clogged with noisy traffic, a woman pulled up and asked for 20 dollars worth of gas. The problem was, Toby couldn't understand what kind of gas she wanted. "She was mumbling and she had her radio on," he recalls.

He kept asking her and she kept answering and he kept not understanding. Finally she lost her temper and yelled, "What are you, deaf?"

"As a matter of fact," Toby replied, "I am."

The woman was so embarrassed she drove off without bothering to fill up. Toby and his fellow pump jockeys got a good laugh out of it. "I mean, what else could you do?"

Given the chance to address a group of parents of newly diagnosed hard-of-hearing children, Toby knows exactly what he'd say: "Be supportive, be patient, be anything a parent would be. Just know your child can do all things. Parents shouldn't feel too bummed or sad or think because their kid has a hearing impairment they won't be able to do anything. I look at myself, and I know a couple of other guys who have hearing aids and are doing quite well for themselves. Anything's possible."

## Danielle

When Danielle was growing up, she used to have scary dreams about the bad things that could happen to her hearing aids. "One time I dreamt that my mom was doing the dishes and I was asking her something, and I dropped them into the sink and I was afraid they would get completely destroyed by water," she recalls.

Nothing bad ever did happen. That's because Danielle, who has a moderate-to-severe loss, took good care of her hearing aids. She'd started wearing them shortly before her 5th birthday when she lost her hearing for reasons that doctors were never able to determine.

"I realized how important they were," she says. "I had already had my hearing. I knew what it was like to hear, and then I couldn't, and after I got my hearing aids I could hear again."

Danielle's hearing aids never did fail her. Less dependable were some of the teachers and administrators she encountered between elementary and high school. Through first grade everyone was supportive and accommodating, but in second grade the teacher refused to use Danielle's FM. The device had been in the repair shop when school began, and by the time it was fixed the teacher was convinced Danielle didn't need it.

"She said Danielle could hear," recalls Danielle's mother, Lillian. A hearing consultant was able to convince the teacher that Danielle needed the device to reach her potential in the classroom, but by then Danielle didn't trust the teacher.

"It took me about 6 months to convince her that every time the teacher did something, it wasn't because she hated her," Lillian says. "The teacher wasn't aware of that—I was dealing with it at home, because I felt if I talked to her about it, it would create more problems."

During the next 11 years, until Danielle graduated from high school in 2005, Lillian often did battle with school officials she felt weren't adequately meeting Danielle's needs. In fifth grade there was a music teacher who refused to wear the boom mike for Danielle's FM because she was afraid it would give her germs. Later that year, the FM was stolen and the family had to replace it because the school refused to buy one. In junior high there was a principal who accused the family of demanding too much.

The school problems began taking a toll on Danielle when she was in junior high. She developed irritable bowel syndrome (IBS), a stress-related illness that compromised her immune system, left her exhausted and bloated, and caused her to miss a significant amount of school.

Aware of her limits, for high school Danielle chose the least stressful program offered by her school district. She could work at her own pace and attend classes infrequently, something she felt would help because the constant class changes and having to always listen through the FM left her fatigued.

Now in college, Danielle is having the most positive educational experience she's had in years. "I've had so much more support," she says. "They have services for students with disabilities, and the woman who runs the program is amazing. She has done everything she could to help me. I've had Communication Access Realtime Translation (CART) providers for the first time in school."

That's not to say there haven't been problems, but Danielle has the poise and self-assurance to handle them. All those years of watching her mother advocate have paid off. "She was always there for me, always supporting me," Danielle says. "As soon as I came home upset, if it was something that meant she needed to talk to someone, she would go do it. That's my mom's personality. I don't think anything that happened could have been avoided or done differently. I think it all would have turned out the way it did eventually, or it would have been worse if she wasn't there."

Hearing loss is described as "an invisible disability," but Danielle doesn't see it that way. "When I'm showing my hearing aids, or in a classroom setting up my FM or giving it to a teacher, I have to stand up straight and be confident," she says.

When she presented her FM boom mike to her college psychology professor the first day of class and the professor turned to the class and announced, "I guess I don't get to have a good hair day," Danielle was determined not to let the professor's attitude demoralize her or make her flee from the class. It helped that her CART provider was supportive and expressed her shock at the inappropriate comment.

After a few days of classes, Danielle realized the professor wasn't the right one for her. She spoke quickly and went through her presentations so rapidly that it was hard for Danielle—and other students—to keep up. "If you asked her to go back so you could finish copying something down, she would say no, she didn't have time. I've been in other professor's classes, and they're willing to do that."

Eventually Danielle transferred to a class with a more accommodating professor. "I wish everyone was like some of my professors," she says. "I just wish they understood that hearing loss is a serious disability and how complex it is, that it's not something that can be fixed just like that. People have to work every day, depending on the severity of their loss, to understand things, or to be in a social situation, or a classroom."

Danielle has made a point of teaching other people about hearing loss. It started in elementary school, when she and her mother did a presentation at the beginning of every school year, to help her classmates understand why she wore hearing aids. More recently she has done presentations at local elementary schools about protecting hearing.

She has no doubt that her skill and comfort with public speaking is a direct result of her past experiences. "I had to start advocating for myself when I was young, and I think that made me more mature," she says. "You're talking to teachers, and you're so many years younger than they are, and you're telling them that they have to do certain things.

"I guess that's one thing that's a positive," she adds. "Another thing I've noticed is that a lot of people have commented that my brothers speak so clearly and they're always considerate with people, talking to teachers and other people. I guess they speak differently than other kids do, because they grew up with me."

When it comes to her hearing loss, focusing on the positive is something that seems to come naturally to Danielle. She says there are things she'd change about her life, but the hearing loss isn't necessarily one of them. "I wish I had never gotten IBS," she says. "I'd rather deal with the hearing loss. Hearing loss is so much more manageable.

"Yeah, I wish that I was 'normal,' but maybe this is what makes me who I am," she adds. "It's built me to who I am now. I like to think that a lot of what I went through in school made me really strong, and made me realize that it could be worse, and I worked through it as much as I could instead of sitting down and feeling sorry for myself. If someone told me that I could have perfect hearing again, I wouldn't say no, but I'm not sorry about my life."

## Katy

Katy was born with normal hearing, but a bout of meningitis just before her 2nd birthday left her with no hearing in one ear and a severe-to-profound loss in the other. The family moved from their farm to Omaha, NE, 400 miles away, so Katy could get the services she'd need to succeed in school and in life.

Katy's parents were adamant about making sure her hearing loss was recognized, and that with a little help, she could be a normal student. They attended her annual IEP meeting, which allowed them to teach her teachers and the school faculty about the accommodations she would need.

"Sometimes I felt embarrassed that I was being earmarked, but looking back I realize how much my parents actually helped me, by doing the things they did," she says. "In restaurants I would make them order for me, to make it less embarrassing when I couldn't understand the waiter or waitress. But around middle school, they started making me do things myself, which helped me to become more independent with my hearing loss."

An A student in high school, Katy majored in psychology at a small competitive liberal arts college in the Midwest. She was captain of the basketball team, which she helped lead to the conference tournament and its first winning season in more than 10 years. She made all-conference 4 years in a row and became the second all-time leading scorer.

Although she had traveled on her own, as far as Japan, college marked the first time Katy had been away from her parents for an extended period of time. It made her realize even more strongly that their intervention made social situations easier for her. "I had always had my mom to rely on in terms of helping me out when I was having trouble hearing," she recalls. "She would go in and talk to all my teachers about my hearing loss. In college, I had to really be active in letting people know when I needed help. That part was really hard for me."

Katy didn't have to fight for accommodations: she simply went to the Academic Advising Disability Services Office and arranged for a note taker and a headset for classes where there were guest speakers. But neither situation was ideal. Katy still had to strain to follow what was happening in class.

"Because of the small class sizes and the types of classes I took, a lot of the classes were discussion based," she says. "There really wasn't anything to help me understand my fellow classmates and I often had to focus very hard to stay in the discussion. But it seems too often that I felt like I had missed quite a bit. It helped me to take classes with my friends, but that didn't always work because I didn't want to have to take classes I didn't have an interest in just because my friends were taking them."

Looking back, Katy wishes Academic Advising had been more proactive. "They only set it up. They didn't follow through and check to see how everything worked out," she says. "It ended up being okay, but they definitely could have done more to help me."

Katy's advice to hard-of-hearing students going to college is "Become your own advocate. No one else is going to do it for you anymore. It took me a couple of semesters to realize that, and then I began trying to reach out and get the help and services I needed."

Trying to decide when to tell people about her hearing loss and when to keep quiet about it has always been a concern for Katy. She doesn't like drawing attention to herself because she doesn't want people to see her as different, so usually she keeps quiet and tries to follow what's being said.

But among the lessons she learned in college was when to speak up for herself. One day a class she was taking broke into small discussion groups and the room suddenly filled with distracting background noise. Katy couldn't make out anything that was being said. She asked that her group be allowed to go into the hall, where it was quiet.

Another tactic she began using is to move to the right of people, situating herself so that her "good" left ear is closer to the sound source. "A lot of my friends have caught on to this and will often help accommodate me and make it easier for me," she says.

"I feel like I have to make the extra effort to make people comfortable, which may be why I don't bring up my hearing right away, because people sometimes get nervous and overarticulate or talk extremely loudly. I generally like to joke about it and talk about it once I get to know people better, to let them know I'm okay with it, and that I'm okay talking about it, so they can feel more comfortable about asking me."

Katy says her hearing loss has forced her to be assertive, but being assertive off the basketball court is not something that comes naturally. There have been many times when she hasn't been able to hear, but has pretended she could.

In classroom situations she'd get frustrated and angry at herself for lacking the courage to speak up when she needed more help hearing. "In conversations with friends, I think I've been doing it for so long I barely realize it anymore," she said a few years ago, when she was in college. "I usually just try to follow as best I can and fill in what I missed, kind of like fill-in-the-blank. The funny thing is, my closest friends realize I do this and they'll stop and say, 'You didn't hear me, did you?' even though I'd been nodding all along. So we laugh about it, and then they fill me in on what I'm missing."

Slowly Katy began gaining the confidence and developing the comfort level to let people know, when necessary, that she's hard of hearing. "I've come to realize that people don't see you as all that different, because what counts most is your personality."

Katy doesn't remember anyone making fun of her because of her hearing loss when she was growing up, but she does recall people saying that her speech sounded "weird." That made her self-conscious about speaking, but she's come to realize that "the more I think about it, the more it hinders me."

The hearing loss also meant she had to work harder to succeed in school, which, she says, was sometimes frustrating. It was also "painful," she says, in places such as a lunchroom or a busy restaurant with background noise.

But Katy comes from a family that tends to dwell on the positive, and over the years her hearing loss has provided a surprising number of opportunities for a good laugh. When she was a child and her parents got mad at her, she knew she'd get a smile if she turned off her aid so she didn't have to listen to them yelling. Once, in a basketball game, she scored two points after her hearing aid tumbled to the floor and everyone in the gym thought her ear had fallen off.

"The ref didn't know what to do, so he just stood there along with everyone else, and I dribbled in for a wide open lay-up."

After graduating from college, Katy moved to Arizona to coach a high school girls' basketball team. She spent a year as a substitute teacher before being hired to teach full time. On the first day of class, she tells students that they need to raise their hands because voice recognition and location are difficult for her.

"They seem to be understanding for the most part," she says. "I have always tried to joke about it, because it lets people know that I'm okay with it and it doesn't need to be the elephant in the room. So I'll occasionally use times when the kids haven't been listening to make a joke."

One day Katy got frustrated when a student wasn't paying attention. She pulled out her hearing aid, offered it to the youngster and said, "Here. I think you need this more than I do."

According to her mom, Dee Ann, Katy has developed extraordinary peripheral vision—something that helps her on the basketball court and in the classroom. She doesn't allow students to text message in class, but they do anyway. And she always catches them. When they ask how, she replies, "I'm deaf, not blind."

During her first year as a teacher, Katy lived with her sister's family. After being hired full time, she moved into an apartment with a roommate. Her only concession to her hearing loss is using her phone as an alarm clock. It vibrates and it's loud, though not as loud as the flashing fire alarm that college officials installed in her dorm room her senior year. "It was the loudest thing I've ever heard," she says. "There was no way I was going to sleep through that."

If she ever moves out on her own, Katy says, she'll look into different technological aids and also a hearing dog. One aid she has no interest in, however, is a cochlear implant. "From my understanding I am not a good candidate," she says. "I hear well enough with my good ear that I can function pretty well in the hearing world. People have told me it would take up to a year for me to get used to hearing with the cochlear implant. Right now, at this point in life, I don't want to do that. I am waiting for the technological advances that will eventually be available that will be better suited for my kind of hearing loss than a cochlear implant."

Living with hearing loss has taught Katy to laugh instead of mope when things don't go her way. "I can turn awkward situations into funny ones by making a joke about it. It's not disrespectful or anything, but I really feel like there is a lot of humor to be found in my hearing loss. And when I think of how much worse it could have been, with meningitis cases killing kids or causing them to be deaf and blind, I realize how lucky I am."

Katy's advice to youngsters growing up today is to learn to adjust and not feel sorry for themselves. "I used to do that sometimes when I was younger—feel sorry for myself, and think how much easier it would be if I could just hear. But it's probably never going to happen, at least for the near future, so there's no use thinking about it. If you think about all the disabilities you could have, hearing loss isn't so bad, so I feel blessed sometimes that my hearing loss is the only thing I really have to deal with. I've had people ask if I'd rather be blind or deaf, and I always reply deaf, because I think sight is one of the most precious things in the world."

## Joan

Joan was diagnosed with a moderately severe hearing loss when she was 2 years old. It was the mid-1940s, and doctors in her native Australia weren't exactly encouraging.

"My mother was simply told, 'Put her away, she will never do anything,'" Joan recalls.

Joan's mother did the opposite: she worked with her daughter every day. Joan didn't have hearing aids—she thinks they may not have been available in rural New South Wales until the early 1950s

—but she had some residual hearing, and between that and her mother's dedication, she learned to speak.

When Joan was 6, she received her first pair of hearing aids. By then she was in school, and even though teachers always sat her in front of the classroom, she still missed what was being said. When she'd ask the child next to her for clarification, the teacher would accuse her of cheating or "trying to disturb," and send her out of the room. Needless to say, she doesn't have pleasant memories of school.

There was little time for extracurricular activities because she had to work on speech with her mother. Her four siblings often grew resentful because their mother had so little time for them. Joan wanted to dance but she couldn't hear the teacher or make sense of the music; she watched the other girls to see what they were doing, and as a result she was always out of step. She dropped out. Then to her delight, as a teenager she discovered a different type of dance she could do, a "Dancing with the Stars" type program, where the music was louder and she had a partner to help with the steps.

Although Joan believes that her hearing loss made her more anxious than her siblings and afraid of things she couldn't control, it also enabled her to take chances "that perhaps hearing kids wouldn't dare to do," most likely because she didn't always understand what she was getting into. Throughout those growing years Joan was forced to discover for herself what worked for her. Though she didn't tell people she had a hearing loss, she gravitated toward those whose voices were easier to understand. Her love of books deepened: by reading she could pick up what she felt she was missing in school or in conversations. She also discovered that she was good at tennis and track and field, sports where her hearing loss didn't seem to pose a problem and where she could excel.

In 1983 Joan moved to North Carolina. Though she had no trouble finding audiologists and hearing aid dispensers to provide services and equipment, she discovered there was little support beyond that for adults dealing with hearing loss in society. There was nowhere to turn for advice on how to keep a job or how to hear in public settings from churches and theaters to restaurants and lectures.

"It was frustrating and isolating," she says.

She made it her mission to help fill the void. She and her husband formed a company, TACSI Assistive Systems, to provide assistive listening systems, notification devices, and support for people with hearing loss, to ensure "barrier-free access in all aspects of everyday living."

Throughout the years Joan has served on national and state boards of government and advocacy organizations for people with hearing loss. She's convinced that children today have it much better than when she was growing up.

"It's okay to have a hearing loss in the educational setting now," she says. "Parents have the help of professionals to understand more clearly their role in guiding their children toward independence, toward finding the middle ground when trying to decide, 'Is this problem because of my child's hearing loss or is this problem a normal part of growing up?'"

Distance education through the Internet for students of all ages has also made a positive difference. No longer does someone with hearing loss have to struggle to hear over noisy students or understand teachers who speak quickly, with their backs to the room, or who walk while talking (all of which make speech-reading difficult).

In the classroom, sound field systems along with FM systems, captioning, and the acceptance of text communication "should give the child with a hearing loss confidence to dream of and eventually pursue a career without restrictions," Joan says.

Where things haven't improved is for adults in social settings and often in the workplace. Although more and more people are being diagnosed with hearing loss and the number is expected to rise, adults don't receive nearly the same support as their younger counterparts.

"What has struck me is that even now, within society, there is still a denial that hearing loss creates a communication issue," Joan says. "Once a child is out on his own, in many ways the 'accepting' world changes."

Joan advises parents to help their older children learn all they can about assistive listening technologies. They may need their own cords to connect their FM systems to a regular amplification or sound field system and know how to set it up and how to troubleshoot. Once they remove their hearing aids or cochlear implant processors, whether at night or to participate in certain activities, they'll have to understand how to be safe in a nonhearing environment—to be as independent as a normal-hearing child.

And, Joan points out, everyone needs a telephone. The challenge for children with hearing loss is to be even more technically savvy than their friends, choosing phones with text, amplification, clarity, and t-coil compatibility. Joan has learned a lot about MP3s and iPods from her grandchildren, and she's convinced that they're great for kids with hearing loss. "A direct connection improves understanding a lot," she says.

In 2003, Joan received a cochlear implant. Three years later, her other ear was implanted. "I'm quickly catching up on what I missed over the years," she says, but the implants and the assistive technology aren't all that have made her life easier.

Becoming involved with Hearing Loss Association of North Carolina helped her grow into what she calls "almost just another hearing person. I believe living with a hearing loss means knowing others with a hearing loss. We share our understanding of the problem, offer support to each other and educate others," she says. "This is a missing piece to the puzzle of hearing loss."

## Maria

Maria was 3 weeks old when her parents learned that she had a severe-to-profound hearing loss. Fitted with her first pair of hearing aids at 4 months, she began working with a teacher of the hearing impaired about 8 months later. When she was older, her parents made flash cards with sentences to use with her. The flash cards helped her learn to listen, which eventually enabled her to shoot to the top of her class at school.

"I pay so much more attention to what is going on around me," she says. "It's really shaped me as a student."

When Maria was 8 years old, paying attention became more of a challenge because her hearing worsened. Doctors diagnosed her with large vestibular aqueduct syndrome (LVAS). They explained to Maria's parents that LVAS often leads to further hearing loss during puberty. Sure enough, when Maria was 13, she woke up one morning to discover that her hearing in her left ear—traditionally her better ear—had worsened significantly.

When Maria had suffered drops in her hearing in the past, doctors had administered steroids. Sometimes the treatment had boosted her hearing, other times it hadn't. This time the specialists knew the drop was so significant that the only thing that would help would be a cochlear implant. Maria was scheduled for surgery around her 14th birthday.

"The hardest part was having it turned on," she recalls. "It hurt the first time I heard everything through the implant, because it was so much louder than through my hearing aid. My dad zipped up a duffle bag and it was so loud it was like it echoed through my head."

Because implants are programmed, or mapped, gradually, the initial range of frequency is quite small. In the first weeks after the mapping began, Maria had trouble discriminating between voices. The phone was a particular problem: often she didn't know whose voice she was hearing. "They almost all sounded the same—all robotic," she says.

As time went on and the range of frequency was expanded, Maria began to hear the differences in people's voices, and she found she preferred what came through the implant to what came through the hearing aid.

"I hear more frequencies," she says. "I hear more sounds. I came into the lobby of a YMCA and I could hear the pop machine humming for the first time in my life."

Bird sounds also made an impression on her. "With my hearing aid alone, I can barely hear them," she says. "Even with a woodpecker, I have to strain to hear it. But now I can hear almost any kind of bird chirping."

At school Maria uses an FM with her hearing aid, but not with the implant. When teachers show movies, they're generally captioned, or else Maria gets to watch them at home where her mother can help if she has trouble hearing the narration. Once a week a teacher consultant comes to check on how things are going. Usually they go well.

Now in her last year of high school, Maria is beginning to look at colleges. Her favorite subjects are English and science, and she's particularly interested in genetics, which she studied one summer at a college-run camp.

She also likes drama, and she's appeared in many shows at her public high school. In "Bye Bye Birdie" she did a dance routine. "I had a partner who went through it with me to make sure I didn't screw up," she says. "It was a lot of fun."

In a show written by her school drama director, she played against type as a goth girl. "To try to get into character, I dressed in black and tried to be dark all week," she recalls. "It shocked everybody in the school. People I didn't know would go up to my friends and ask what had happened to me."

Maria has a good group of friends at school. If they go out to a restaurant, where it's noisy and hard for her to hear, they'll sit in a quiet area. "Generally my friends are helpful and try to make sure I'm having fun, too," she says. "They've forgotten I'm hearing impaired, and they don't think about it. I do, when I'm in a situation where I need to hear. It's a part of me."

Among the accommodations Maria has at home are captioning on her telephone and television, and a shake-awake alarm clock. Recently, a movie theater in a neighboring town introduced "rear window" captioning, which allows her to read movie captions on a sheet of Plexiglas attached to her cupholder.

To Maria, captions are an unexpected benefit of having a hearing loss. "I like reading, and seeing the captions and being introduced to new words," she says, adding that the captions have helped her to become a good speller.

Another benefit of hearing loss: reading lips. "I like the power of being able to read lips," she says. "People are always fascinated by it."

Lipreading came naturally to Maria. Her parents encouraged her to look at people when they were speaking, because it would help her to pay attention. She's grateful to her parents for all they've done for her, but especially for insisting that she learn to speak and listen.

"It makes me able to participate in the hearing world, which is what the majority of the population is," she says. "My parents have been with me every step of the way, and helped me deal with my hearing loss. That's basically why I'm a good advocate for myself. I would advise other parents to do the best they can and hope for the best. You learn to live with hearing loss, and accept what it is—and maybe even enjoy it."

## David

A math professor at Howard University in Washington, DC, David lost his hearing after contracting meningitis. His diagnosis: profound bilateral hearing loss. But because he could detect some low frequencies in his left ear, his parents had him fitted with a hearing aid. It was 1955 and David was almost 5 years old. His hearing aid consisted of a "box" strapped to his chest and connected by a wire to an earmold and receiver.

"I refused to wear it until my mother took me around to several families on our block in Chicago and had me show them my new device," he recalls. "They cheered and congratulated me on having it. This made it, if nothing else, a symbol of my ties to the community and motivated me to wear it faithfully. Wearing it pretty much all my waking hours for the next several years gave me a chance to learn to use my amplified residual hearing. Ever since, I've worn a hearing aid because it's so much less difficult to understand people when I do."

Understanding is David's biggest challenge, what he considers the greatest drawback to hearing loss. "It takes a lot of work and often can't be done anyway. I can't hear my children talking to each other. Foreign languages, even ones I can read and write, are impossible for me to speak or understand when spoken. One of my brothers is a professional actor: I can appreciate his body language, but not his voice. Deafness *is* a negative thing that cuts me off from a lot of good stuff."

It also had a direct effect on his siblings, all but one of whom were born after David lost his hearing. "Each of them learned how to speak to me while learning how to speak in the first place, and each became consciously aware, at about age 4, that my hearing was limited."

David doesn't think his siblings resented his hearing loss, but he also doesn't deny that it greatly shaped his early relationship with the brother who is closest to his age. Two years old when David became deaf, "he surely did not get as much of our parents' attention as he should have because they were distracted by my crisis, which shadows his earliest memories," David recalls.

The two attended a Catholic elementary school in a rough neighborhood far from theirs, the only school that was willing to accommodate David's disability. "He knew I wasn't aware of many things because I couldn't hear them happening or developing, and he felt responsible for me. That was a serious burden at such a young age. But for all the others, I was a revered big brother."

It wasn't until he was 7 or 8 that David was able to understand people to a useful degree, and only if they were speaking directly to him, facing him, in good light, without too much background noise, and while he was giving them his full attention.

"Even then I can fail to understand," he says, "but under such circumstances it's usually pretty evident from my responses whether I'm getting it or not."

A bigger problem is that people don't and often can't realize that what they're saying directly to him is all he can understand, that he doesn't hear the many other things normal-hearing people do.

"I don't hear what people across the dinner table from me say to each other. I don't overhear. I don't hear things addressed to the group in general, unless I happen to be in the right location at the right time, so it's as if they were addressed directly to me," he says. "I seldom even hear my name called if someone's trying to get my attention. Normal-hearing people hear these things and much more, a lot of which I'm probably not even aware of. They take what they hear for granted, and assume that I do, too, an assumption so unconscious that the conscious knowledge that I'm deaf often does not affect it. Indeed, since people with normal hearing are *always* hearing sounds—ears can't be closed the way eyes can—the very concept of *not* hearing, deafness, can be quite hard to imagine in any concrete, useful, way."

Telling people about his hearing loss isn't an issue for David— if they don't notice his hearing aid, they can usually tell because it's obvious he isn't following the conversation. The bigger issue is whether to call special attention to it. In general, he does that only when he needs accommodations: for example, a particular seat at a lunch table or in a lecture hall so that he can lip-read.

He tells his students at the first class meeting, right after announcing his office location and hours and exam and grading policies. "I inform the class that I'm deaf, I lip-read, and I don't hear my name called so that to ask questions they must raise their hands," he says.

For most students, and most people in general, he says, his deafness is "strictly a practical matter: They just want me to be able to communicate with them reasonably effectively, to understand the questions they ask and answer them usefully and without too much unusual effort."

Raising hands in class is acceptable; having to write out questions probably wouldn't be, he says.

Several times during his teaching career, students have tried to blame their failing grades on David's deafness. It's never worked. "Since other students in the same classes, not to mention the students in my other classes, had no such problems, the departmental chair—and it was a different one each time, as I recall—was completely unsympathetic to the complaining students."

Having a teacher who can't hear you whisper and whose insistence that you remain quiet during lectures and raise a hand before speaking can also prove to be motivating, as it did for at least one of David's students. "After struggling very hard but managing to get an A in the end, he came to my office and said, 'I knew you learned that stuff without even being able to hear it. I could hear it. I had no excuse not to learn it.' "

It would be nice, David says, if more people understood what he calls "the ambiguity of damaged or absent hearing, how it cannot be overcome by simply increasing the volume, how it imposes something analogous to foggy tunnel vision, but also how, if you've lived with it for a long time you've probably learned to deal with it."

David sometimes encounters people who are more sensitive to hearing loss, who seem to genuinely understand how he misses much of what the hearing world hears. "Some of these people fear that I suffer over it, such as by feeling left out," he says. "In fact, I feel I'm living quite a satisfactory life with what I do get."

## Stephanie

When Stephanie, 43, was 5 years old, her mother took her to the audiologist. The appointment was for Stephanie's younger brother Daniel, 2½. Their older sister, Andrea, had been diagnosed several years earlier with a moderate-to-severe loss and their mother was concerned that Daniel was exhibiting similar behavior.

At the time siblings weren't routinely tested, but after Daniel was diagnosed with a moderately severe loss, the audiologist asked to test Stephanie as well.

"My mother assured them she had no concerns about my hearing, but said they could go ahead," Stephanie says. "Imagine her surprise when the results revealed I had a moderate hearing loss. My brother and I got hearing aids the same year—we had the same model body aid that we wore in a harness, under our clothes."

Stephanie and her siblings attended public school in a small town in central Massachusetts. Their primary accommodation was that they always sat in the front row. Their only other assistance consisted of some notes from the audiologist with suggestions about how to help a child with hearing loss function in the classroom: Face the child when speaking, wear red lipstick to make lipreading visible, do not give oral exams (with the exception of spelling tests), and provide a script when filmstrips are shown during class.

"I can recall some funny moments in school trying to sit in the back of class and eventually getting 'reassigned' to a front row seat, even though I had a straight A average in the class," Stephanie recalls. "I was secretly frustrated I was never chosen to advance the film-strips; the teachers were probably afraid I would not hear the 'beep' indicating it was time."

Like her siblings, Stephanie never publicized her hearing loss. It wasn't so much that they were ashamed, she says, it was more "for our own personal vanity. I'm not sure it's as big a deal nowadays, with all the other types of listening devices people wear on their ears, but in the 1970s and 1980s, we were definitely the different kids in our school."

Stephanie served on school committees and played sports. "There was the horrifying moment when I was playing basketball in high school and I got hit in the head and my hearing aid went flying off. I thought no one knew I wore hearing aids, so I was just mortified that I had to pick it up off the floor. I thought everyone was watching me, including my secret crush. I wanted to just melt. But I needed my hearing aid, so I picked it up and went on to play the game. No one ever said a word to me about what happened, so the horror of it was probably magnified in my own head."

Stephanie's parents instilled in her and her siblings that they could do whatever they set their minds to, "that we just needed to work hard, study hard and good things would follow. They definitely did not 'give us a break' because we were hard of hearing. They also never made us feel ashamed that we had hearing loss."

All three were members of the National Honor Society and went on to college. At Boston College, Stephanie studied business and marketing. Her plan was to become an bookkeeper, but her senior honors thesis changed that. Her topic, inspired after she learned that many people who needed hearing aids didn't wear them, was how hearing aids were marketed. She offered recommendations to the industry on how to change their marketing strategies to reach more consumers.

Her thesis advisor was so impressed he tried to dissuade her from going into bookkeeping. "He thought I could make a big impact in the field of hearing health care," she recalls, but she already had a bookkeeping job lined up.

During her year as a bookkeeper, Stephanie thought often about the conversation with her advisor. Finally she sent resumes and cover letters to nearly 20 hearing aid companies, telling them she had unique ideas. She got one phone interview, "which was not the best way for me to represent myself," and one face-to-face interview. Neither company offered her a job. The problem: she lacked the technical background needed to work in the industry.

Stephanie set up a meeting with her audiologist to ask how to get the technical background. "You need a master's degree in audiology," the woman said, but she wasn't exactly encouraging. "She did not know how I would complete the clinical requirements with my hearing loss," Stephanie recalls.

Frustrated, Stephanie shelved the idea and kept working in different business environments. She was not comfortable using the phone, but she was an excellent typist. So she struck deals with coworkers: they'd make her phone calls and she'd do their typing. As a sales representative, she truly pounded the pavement, opting to door-knock rather than make phone calls. Each job lasted about 2 years and each time one ended she'd think back to her conversation with the Boston College advisor.

In 1994, after she and her husband moved to North Carolina, she decided to go to graduate school. The University of North Carolina at Chapel Hill had a graduate program in audiology. Stephanie spoke to the program director, sharing her vision, resume, and transcript from college. For the first time, she was encouraged, as the director told her something she never thought she would hear.

"He said, 'We need more people like you in the field of audiology. I believe we can find a way around the hearing issues.'"

For Stephanie, the first step was learning, for the first time, about FM. The technology made her graduate school experience far easier than her college years. "I used the FM system to hear clients in the clinic and to hear my professors in class; all willingly wore the transmitter," she says. "I was 30 years old before I realized it was okay to tell people I had hearing loss. I always limited how much I told people—fudging my way through things, albeit pretty successfully. However, I learned that it was easier to just let people know what they needed to do. Most people want to communicate with you, but you need to help them understand how they can do it best."

When Stephanie entered graduate school her goal was to get a job in the marketing department of a major hearing aid company. But after she began seeing patients as part of her course work, she realized she had found her calling.

After completing the graduate program, Stephanie took a job with an audiologist in private practice. Occasionally the owner of the practice or a colleague needed to help her determine if a patient's hearing aid was squealing or if it sounded distorted, but most of the time she worked independently. She enjoyed working with patients and her patients loved working with her because they knew she understood hearing loss. Her network of people with hearing loss grew through her work at the clinic and at the local Self-Help for the Hard of Hearing group, now called Hearing Loss Association of America. She was a professional advisor for the group and made many friends there.

In 1999, Stephanie returned to UNC-Chapel Hill as a visiting instructor, and began to pursue her doctorate in audiology. In 2001, she was approached by the director of UNC's Speech and Hearing Sciences Division, the professor who had encouraged her years earlier to pursue her first audiology degree, to apply for the position of clinic coordinator. It was the perfect marriage of her job and life experiences. She could use her business skills, work with patients, and help teach the next generation of audiologists.

"I find being a professor of audiology extremely rewarding," she says. "I enjoy teaching and giving my students the perspective of what it's like for the person or family sitting on the other side of our equipment. I am candid with my students concerning my feelings about being hard of hearing. For me, most of the time, I just feel like a person who sometimes does not hear well. I have never felt 'disabled' and have done everything I have ever set out to do. Maybe I'm a Pollyanna who always sees the glass as half full. I always try to find a lesson and a way to grow from everything I have ever experienced in my life, and try to find a way to use it to benefit others."

Stephanie has been married for almost 17 years and has two sons under 5 years old. Her husband and children all have normal hearing. Her sons learned as soon as they could walk that before they could talk to Mommy in the morning, they had to give her the hearing aids on her nightstand. When she and her husband are apart they keep in touch with e-mail and instant messaging.

"Technology today makes communication so much easier than ever before," she says. "The captioning is always on the TV if I come in the room. Sure, there are moments of frustration, but that's normal in any relationship, not just with those who have hearing loss."

Over the years, Stephanie and her siblings continued to lose hearing until all three had profound losses. Genetic testing has shown that they have a mutation of otoferlin, but researchers are still searching for a second, deafness-causing gene. "There was definitely some comfort for us in knowing what caused our hearing loss, but none of us have gotten overly caught up in it," Stephanie says.

In 1999, Stephanie's brother, Daniel, visited her and attended a class she was teaching at UNC on cochlear implants. The experience made such an impact on him that he decided to get an implant.

"He now can talk to just about anyone on the phone and it has changed his whole world," Stephanie says. "He serves as a patient liaison for one of the cochlear implant companies, traveling to conferences and chatting on-line with potential cochlear implant candidates to help them make informed decisions about implantation for themselves or their child."

Stephanie is now preparing to get an implant herself. The implant team at UNC is encouraged because of Daniel's progress and they believe she, too, is a good candidate. "I know getting the cochlear implant now is going to make a big difference for the next chapter of my life," she says. "I feel blessed that I have been able to use my life experiences in a positive way, and look forward to continuing to do so. I think it's easy for parents to get wrapped up thinking about all the things their child might not be able to do when they find out about the hearing loss, but we have come so far in the 40-plus years since my sister was diagnosed with hearing loss. I believe the future will only get brighter as technology continues to improve, and as we focus more and more on auditory training and communication strategies. And as a growing number of young people pursue audiology as a profession, we will have an even greater number of compassionate audiologists working with families and children who have hearing loss."

## Conclusion

The personal stories shared by adults provide valuable insight on how hearing loss impacts life in ways not easily comprehended by professionals or even parents. But it's important to remember that each person's experiences are different. Moreover, the stories our children will tell as adults may be quite different. For families who choose spoken language as a primary means of communication, and whose children have access to early identification, early diagnosis, modern hearing technology, and appropriate intervention services, congenital hearing loss doesn't mean what it once did. For many children, with appropriate hearing technology and competent professional services, it is possible to achieve successful auditory-oral communication even with profound deafness. Indeed, many children with congenital hearing loss today have difficulty qualifying for special services at school. Our challenge now is to make the best possible resources available to all families. This requires a partnership of parents and professionals, working together as advocates to ensure that the stories of tomorrow are not about deafness but about the choices available to all children.

# AFTERWORD

In the 10 years since Elizabeth began wearing hearing aids, our family life has changed more than I could have imagined. I realize the same can be said by any parent over the course of 10 years, regardless of her child's hearing. But what's taken me by surprise is that as I was researching this book and learning more about pediatric hearing loss and how to help children and families affected by it, my daily responsibilities regarding Elizabeth's hearing were diminishing.

By the time she was 7 years old I no longer had to remove her hearing aids every night and clean and test them in the morning. She took them off before bed and cleaned them. In the morning she put them in. I still keep fresh batteries in a case on my key chain, but she carries spares to school and soccer practice. When a battery dies, she changes it, even if I'm the one with the extras. When her ears feel waxy, she wipes them with a damp cloth.

The same won't necessarily hold true for every child. Some become independent earlier. Others, for whom hearing loss is part of a larger spectrum of health problems or developmental delays, may never become fully independent. Regardless of your child's situation, though, the one thing you can count on is that nothing will remain static.

What Jack and I hope we've done here is provide you with a useful introduction to the world of hearing loss in children. As your child grows, needs will change and, as a result, so will your responsibilities. There will be pieces you'll still have to put together, but as we've shown here, there are many people and organizations to help you along the way. We wish you the best in this journey.

# GLOSSARY

**Acute otitis media:** An infection of the middle ear that often includes pain, fever, and conductive hearing loss.

**Air conduction pathway:** The transmission of sound through the outer and middle ear to the cochlea.

**Air conduction threshold:** The hearing threshold for a pure-tone stimulus delivered from an earphone or insert receiver.

**American Academy of Audiology (AAA):** A national professional association of audiologists.

**American Speech-Language-Hearing Association (ASHA):** A national professional association of audiologists, speech-language pathologists, and speech, hearing, and language scientists.

**Amplification:** An increase in the intensity of sounds provided by a hearing aid.

**Analog (hearing aid):** A type of hearing aid that provides amplification by continuous changes in sound processing.

**Audiogram:** Graphic representation of hearing thresholds plotted on a chart to show the softest tone a person can detect at various frequencies from low pitch to high pitch.

**Audiologist:** A health care professional whose professional practices include prevention, evaluation, and rehabilitation of hearing impairment and related disorders.

**Auditory brainstem response (ABR):** Neurological responses produced by the auditory nerve and brainstem in response to sound. Audiologists use ABRs to screen for hearing loss, to estimate hearing threshold levels, and to evaluate processing at the level of the auditory nerve and brainstem.

**Auditory neuropathy:** A hearing disorder that causes difficulty understanding speech and other sounds because of a disturbance in the transmission of signals from the inner ear to the brain. The condition has also been called *auditory dys-synchrony*. It usually affects both ears. Because the characteristics are so variable some experts have recommended the term *auditory neuropathy spectrum disorder*.

**Auditory processing disorder:** A disorder of auditory processing resulting from disease, trauma, or abnormal development of the auditory system.

**Behavioral hearing tests:** Assessment procedures involving observable responses to sound.

**Bilateral hearing loss:** Reduction of hearing sensitivity in both ears.

**Binaural hearing:** Hearing with both ears.

**Bone conduction:** A hearing test that involves transmitting sound to the inner ear using a small vibrator applied to the skull.

**CART:** Communication Access Realtime Translation (CART) is a live captioning service for the deaf and hard of hearing that provides a visual display of everything that is said, usually on a screen or monitor, for meetings and conferences.

**Cerumen:** Substance secreted from glands in the ear canal, commonly referred to as *earwax*.

**Cochlea:** Auditory portion of the inner ear, consisting of fluid-filled channels that contain hair cell receptors.

**Cochlear implant:** A hearing device that consists of an electrode array surgically implanted in the cochlea. It delivers electrical signals to the auditory nerve from an external processor, enabling people with severe-to-profound hearing loss to perceive sound.

**Conductive hearing loss:** Reduction in hearing sensitivity due to reduced sound transmission resulting from abnormality of the external ear canal, eardrum, or middle ear.

**Digital (hearing aid):** A type of hearing aid that provides amplification by changing the incoming sound into streams of data.

**Ear infection:** See acute otitis media and otitis externa.

**Earmold:** A custom-fitted device to deliver sound from a behind-the-ear hearing aid into the ear canal. It also helps to hold the hearing aid in place.

**Eustachian tube:** The passageway leading from throat to the middle ear; it opens during yawning and swallowing to equalize middle ear air pressure.

**Frequency:** Also known as Hertz (Hz), it is the number of cycles occurring in one second. It corresponds to a listener's perception of pitch.

**Hair cells:** Sensory cells in the inner ear where nerve endings attach to the auditory nerve.

**Hearing level (HL):** The decibel level of sound as it relates to normal hearing.

**Masking noise:** Sounds used by audiologists to prevent one ear from hearing while the other is being tested.

**Meningitis:** A bacterial or viral infection that can cause auditory disorders due to infection or inflammation of the inner ear or auditory nerve.

**Mixed hearing loss:** Hearing loss with both conductive and sensorineural components.

**Objective test procedures:** Measurement of hearing sensitivity based on estimates made from physiologic responses to sound. Examples include auditory brainstem responses (ABR) and otoacoustic emissions (OAE).

**Otitis externa:** Inflammation of the ear canal. It may be accompanied by pain, swelling, and secretions.

**Otitis media (OM):** Inflammation of the middle ear.

**Otitis media with effusion (OME):** Inflammation of the middle ear with an accumulation of fluid behind the eardrum in the middle ear space.

**Otoacoustic emissions (OAE):** Low-level sounds produced by the cochlea and measured by audiologists to evaluate inner ear (cochlear) function.

**Otolaryngologist:** A physician who specializes in the diagnosis and treatment of diseases of the ear, nose, and throat, including diseases of related structures of the head and neck.

**Otoscope:** An optical device that provides light and magnification for the visual examination of the ear canal and eardrum.

**Ototoxic:** Medications potentially harmful to the auditory system.

**Pure tone:** A single frequency used by audiologists to evaluate hearing sensitivity.

**Pure-tone air conduction audiometry:** Measurement of hearing for pure-tone sounds and speech presented through earphones, insert receivers, or a loudspeaker.

**Pure-tone audiometer:** An instrument for presenting pure tones of different frequencies and intensities.

**Pure-tone bone conduction audiometry:** Measurement of hearing thresholds to pure-tone sounds presented from a small vibrator placed against the skull.

**Pure-tone screening:** Test used to screen for hearing loss at a fixed level, typically 20 dB HL.

**Pure-tone threshold audiometry:** Determination of the lowest level a pure tone can be detected about 50% of the time.

**Recessive genetic condition:** An inherited condition in which both parents carry an abnormal gene. For each pregnancy there is a 25% chance the child will be affected.

**Residual hearing:** The amount of functional hearing available to a person with a sensorineural hearing loss.

**Rubella:** A viral infection characterized by fever and skin rash that resembles measles; may result in abnormalities in the unborn child including sensorineural hearing loss (also known as *German measles*).

**Sensorineural hearing loss:** Loss of hearing sensitivity due to disorders involving the cochlea and/or the auditory nerve.

**Serous otitis media:** Inflammation of the middle ear with an accumulation of thin, watery (serous) fluid.

**Signal-to-noise ratio:** The relationship of a primary signal to the level of background noise. People with hearing loss need a *better* signal-to-noise ratio than people with normal hearing.

**Sound bore:** A channel through the earmold where sound passes through the earmold tubing to the ear canal.

**Speech-language pathologist:** Health care professional whose professional practice includes evaluation, rehabilitation, and prevention of speech and language disorders.

**Speech reception threshold:** Determination of the lowest level speech can be understood about 50% of the time; testing is usually conducted using two-syllable (spondee) words.

**Threshold:** In audiometry, the softest sounds (usually pure tones or speech) a person can detect.

**Tympanic membrane:** A thin membrane at the end of the ear canal that vibrates in response to incoming sounds. The vibrations are transmitted to the middle and inner ear.

**Tympanogram:** A graph that shows how well the eardrum and middle ear respond to sound; can be used to identify middle ear disorders requiring medical attention.

**Tympanometer:** Instrument used to detect middle ear disorders such as otitis media.

**Tympanostomy tube:** Small tube inserted in the eardrum by an otolaryngologist to equalize air pressure in the middle ear; also known as a *pressure equalization* (PE) tube.

**Unilateral hearing loss:** Loss of hearing sensitivity in one ear only.

# RECOMMENDED READINGS

It's not always easy to find books about hearing loss in children. Local bookstores may carry one or two titles, but I've found that the best place to look is the Alexander Graham Bell Web site. (The address is listed in the Resources section.) The following list, while by no means comprehensive, includes books that some of my parenting friends and I have found particularly helpful.

Candlish, P. A. M. (1996). *Not deaf enough: Raising a child who is hard of hearing.* Washington, DC: Alexander Graham Bell Association for the Deaf and Hard of Hearing.

Davis, J. M. (Ed.). (2001). *Our forgotten children: Hard of hearing pupils in the schools* (3rd ed.). Bethesda, MD: Self Help for Hard of Hearing People Publications.

Luterman, D., & Ross, M. (1991). *When your child is deaf: A guide for parents.* Baltimore: York Press.

Safer, J. (2003). *The normal one: Life with a difficult or damaged sibling.* New York: Delta.

Schwartz, S. (1996). *Choices in deafness: A parents' guide to communication options.* Bethesda, MD: Woodbine House.

Tucker, B. P. (1997). *Idea advocacy for children who are deaf or hard of hearing.* San Diego, CA: Singular.

Wayner, D. (2001). *Hearing and learning: A guide to helping children.* Austin, TX: Hear Again.

Wayner, D. S., & Rupert, E. I. (2001). *Voices from a quieter land: Insights into the impact of hearing impairment.* Austin, TX: Hear Again.

Wright, P., & Wright, M. (2002). *Wrightslaw: From emotions to advocacy —The special education survival guide.* Hatfield, VA: Harbor House Law Press.

# RESOURCES

**Advanced Bionics Corporation:** http://www.cochlearimplant
.com Link to Advanced Bionics Web site to learn about its cochlear implants. This Web site contains some technical information and a good section on frequently asked questions.

25129 Rye Canyon Loop
Valencia, CA 91355
(877) 829-0026

**Alexander Graham Bell Association for the Deaf and Hard of Hearing (AG Bell):** http://www.agbell.org The Alexander Graham Bell Association for the Deaf and Hard of Hearing is one of the world's largest membership organizations and information centers on hearing loss and the auditory approach. AG Bell promotes the use of spoken language by children and adults with hearing loss. Through advocacy, publications, financial aid and scholarships, and numerous programs and services, AG Bell promotes its mission: Advocating Independence through Listening and Talking!

3417 Volta Place, NW
Washington, DC 20007
(202) 337-5220

**American Academy of Audiology:** http://www.audiology.org With more than 10,000 members, the American Academy of Audiology (AAA) is the world's largest professional organization of, for, and by audiologists. The AAA promotes quality hearing and balance care for adults and children by advancing the profession of

audiology through leadership, advocacy, education, public awareness, and support of research.

11730 Plaza America Drive, Suite 300
Reston, VA 20190
(800) AAA-2336

**American Academy of Otolaryngology-Head and Neck Surgery:**
http://www.entnet.org The Academy represents more than 12,000
otolaryngologist-head and neck surgeons who diagnose and treat
disorders of the ears, nose, throat, and related structures of the
head and neck.

1650 Diagonal Road
Alexandria, VA 22314
(703) 836-4444

**AAP Champion Initiative:** http://www.aap.org The American
Academy of Pediatrics' hearing screening initiative is designed to
improve the quality of newborn hearing screening, diagnosis, and
intervention programs by increasing the appropriate involvement
of primary care pediatricians and other physicians who care for
children and by linking follow-up services more closely to the
newborn's medical home, as defined by the Joint Committee on
Infant Hearing.

The American Academy of Pediatrics
141 Northwest Point Boulevard
Elk Grove Village, IL 60007-1098
(847) 434-4000

**American Association of the Deaf-Blind:** http://www.aadb.org/
The American Association of the Deaf-Blind (AADB) is a national
consumer advocacy organization for people who have combined
hearing and vision impairments.

8630 Fenton Street, Suite 121
Silver Springs, MD 20910
(301) 495-4403

**American Society for Deaf Children (ASDC):** http://www.deaf
children.org ASDC's primary mission is to advocate for the high-

est quality programs and services for parents so they are able to make reasoned and informed choices to meet their children's educational, communication, personal, and social needs.

800 Florida Avenue NE, #2047
Washington, DC 20002-3695
(800) 942-2732 (Parent Hotline)

**American Speech-Language-Hearing Association (ASHA):** http://www.asha.org   ASHA's mission is to ensure that all people with speech, language, and hearing disorders have access to quality services to help them communicate more effectively. ASHA's Web site also contains a directory of audiologists and speech pathologists.

2200 Research Boulevard
Rockville, MD 20850
(301) 296-5700

**BEGINNINGS for Parents of Children Who Are Deaf or Hard of Hearing, Inc.:** http://www.ncbegin.org   BEGINNINGS for Parents of Children Who are Deaf or Hard of Hearing, Inc. was established in 1987 to provide emotional support and access to information for families with deaf or hard of hearing children up to age 21. The organization provides an impartial approach to meeting the diverse needs of these families and the professionals who serve them. (These services are also available to deaf parents who have hearing children.) The mission of BEGINNINGS is to help parents be informed, empowered, and supported as they make decisions about their child. The BEGINNINGS Web site, which serves families and professionals, includes topics such as early intervention, communication options, audiology and assistive technology, and school issues.

P.O. Box 17646
Raleigh, NC 27619
(919) 850-2746

**Canadian Academy of Audiology:** http://www.canadianaudiology.ca   The Canadian Academy of Audiology is a professional organization dedicated to enhancing the profession of audiology, and providing quality hearing health care and education to those with, or at risk for, hearing and/or vestibular disorders. The academy further strives to represent the audiological community on relevant national issues in a timely, organized manner.

> 1771 Avenue Road
> P.O. Box 54541
> Toronto, ON M5M 4N5
> (905) 319-6191 / (800) 264-5106

**Canadian Association of Speech-Language Pathologists and Audiologists (CASLPA):** http://www.caslpa.ca   With over 5,000 members, CASLPA is the single national body that supports the needs, interests, and development of speech-language pathologists and audiologists across Canada.

> 1 Nicholas Street, Suite 100
> Ottawa, ON K1N 7B7
> (613) 567-9968 / (800) 259-8519

**The Canadian Hard of Hearing Association:** http://www .chha.ca   The Canadian Hard of Hearing Association (CHHA) is a consumer-based organization formed in 1982 by and for hard-of-hearing Canadians. CHHA works cooperatively with professionals, service providers, and government bodies and provides information about hard of hearing issues and solutions. CHHA is the national voice of hard-of-hearing Canadians. It provides a vehicle for hard-of-hearing and deafened people to make their needs known, and to work at ensuring that those needs are identified and addressed. The philosophy of CHHA is to produce knowledgeable hard-of-hearing consumers who understand how to have their needs met. Its mission is to raise public awareness concerning issues that are important for persons who are hard of hearing, to promote their integration in Canadian society, to remove any barriers to their participation, and to generally make every community in Canada a better place for people who are hard of hearing.

> 2415 Holly Lane
> Suite 205
> Ottawa, ON K1V 7P2
> (613) 526-1584

**The Canadian Hearing Society:** http://www.chs.ca The Canadian Hearing Society provides services that enhance the independence of deaf, deafened, and hard-of-hearing people, and that encourage prevention of hearing loss.

271 Spadina Road
Toronto, ON M5R 2V3
(877) 347 3427

**Center for Hearing Loss in Children, Boys Town National Research Hospital:** http://www.boystownhospital.org/home.asp The Boys Town National Research Hospital is a nationally-oriented clinical and research facility dedicated to the study and treatment of children's communication disorders. The efforts of the Hospital's multidisciplinary staff are closely coordinated with the programs of the Center for Hearing Loss in Children.

Boys Town National Research Hospital
555 N. 30th Street
Omaha, NE 68131
(402) 498-6511

**Centers for Disease Control and Prevention (CDC):** http://www.cdc.gov/ncbddd/ehdi/ The CDC, through its Early Hearing Detection and Intervention (EHDI) Program, maintains an informative website for parents and professionals. Educational materials of interest to parents are available on line and by mail order.

Centers for Disease Control and Prevention
1600 Clifton Rd.
Atlanta, GA 30333
(800) 232-4636

**Cochlear Corporation:** http://www.cochlearamericas.com/ This is a link to the Cochlear Corporation Web site, which allows parents to learn more about Cochlear's different cochlear implants. The site contains highly technical information and a more accessible section on recipients and their stories.

Cochlear Americas
13059 E. Peakview Avenue
Centennial, CO 80111
(800) 523-5798

**Council for Exceptional Children:** http://www.cec.sped.org
The Council for Exceptional Children (CEC) is an international professional organization dedicated to improving educational outcomes for individuals including students with disabilities and/or the gifted. CEC advocates for appropriate governmental policies, sets professional standards, provides continual professional development, advocates for newly and historically underserved individuals with "exceptionalities," and helps professionals obtain conditions and resources necessary for effective professional practice.

1110 North Glebe Road, Suite 300
Arlington, VA 22201-5704
(888) 232-7733
TTY: (866) 915-5000 (text only)

**Deafness Research Foundation:** http://www.drf.org   The Deafness Research Foundation (DRF) is the leading national source of private funding for basic and clinical research in hearing science. The DRF is committed to making lifelong hearing health a national priority by funding research and implementing education projects in both the government and private sectors.

641 Lexington Avenue FI 15
New York, NY 10022
(866) 454-3924
TTY: (888) 435-6104

**The Deaf Resource Library:** http://www.deaflibrary.org   The Deaf Resource Library is a virtual library, an on-line collection of reference material and links intended to educate and inform people about Deaf cultures in Japan and the United States, as well as deaf and hard of hearing related topics.

**Described and Captioned Media Program:** http://www.dcmp .org   This free-loan media and open-captioned program is funded by the U.S. Department of Education. People who are deaf or hard-of-hearing persons, teachers, parents, and others may borrow materials without having to pay rental, postage, or registration fees. Other services include free information about captioning and assistance to captioning companies on request.

Described and Captioned Media Program
National Association of the Deaf
1447 E. Main Street
Spartanburg, SC 29307
(800) 237-6213

**Educational Audiology Association:** http://www.edaud.org
The Educational Audiology Association (EAA) is an international
organization of audiologists and related professionals who deliver a
full spectrum of hearing services to all children, particularly those
in educational settings. The mission of EAA is to act as the primary
resource and active advocate for its members through its publications and products, continuing educational activities, networking
opportunities, and other professional endeavors.

3030 W. 81st Avenue
Westminster, CO 80031-4111
(800) 460-7322

**The Electronic Deaf Education Network (EDEN):** http://www
.bradingrao.com/   A comprehensive and informative Web site developed and maintained by Brad Ingrao, an audiologist whose son
is deaf, EDEN offers parents support, ideas, and information from
a variety of sources with a wealth of knowledge about how to help
children who are hard of hearing or deaf. The Web site also has
a chatroom and a library.

**Hands & Voices:** http://www.handsandvoices.org   Hands & Voices
is a parent-driven, nonprofit organization dedicated to providing
unbiased support to families with children who are deaf or hard of
hearing. Programs and activities for parents and professionals may
include outreach events, educational seminars, advocacy, lobbying
efforts, parent–to-parent networking, and a newsletter. Hands &
Voices also strives to connect families with resources and information to make informed decisions around the issues of deafness or
hearing loss.

P.O. Box 3093
Boulder, CO 80307
(303) 492-6283

**Hearing Ear Dogs of Canada:** http://www.dogguides.com/pro grams/programs03.htm   The Lions Foundation of Canada trains dog guides to meet the needs of Canadians with hearing and other medically and physically limiting disabilities. All programs are offered at no charge to the client, but future care and maintenance become the responsibility of the dog guide recipient.

> P.O. Box 907
> Oakville, ON L6J 5E8
> (800) 768-3030

**The Hearing Exchange:** http://www.hearingexchange.com   The Hearing Exchange is an online community for exchanging ideas and information on hearing loss. This site is a useful tool for parents of a child who is hard of hearing or deaf, or for a professional who works with children or adults. No matter what method of communication the family has chosen, they will likely find interesting and supportive information at this site.

> P.O. Box 689
> Jericho, NY 11753
> (516) 938-5475

**Hearing Loss Association of America:** http://www.hearingloss .org   HLA is the nation's largest organization for people with hearing loss. The organization exists to open the world of communication for people with hearing loss through information, education, advocacy, and support. This Web site contains information about state and local chapters in the United States.

**The Hearing Foundation of Canada:** http://www.hearingfoun dation.ca   The Hearing Foundation of Canada is a national charitable organization established in 1979, led by a volunteer board of directors drawn from the business and medical communities, many of whom have personal experience with hearing loss. This organization is committed to eliminating the devastating effects of hearing loss on the quality of life of Canadians, particularly youth, by promoting prevention, early diagnosis, leading-edge medical research, and successful intervention.

> 80 Richmond Street West, Suite 1401
> Toronto, ON M5H 2A4
> (866) 432-7968

**The House Ear Institute:** http://www.hei.org   The House Ear Institute is a nonprofit 501(c)(3) organization dedicated to advancing hearing science through research and education. Institute scientists investigate hearing loss and ear disease as well as the complex neurological interactions between the auditory system and brain. They are also working to improve hearing aids and auditory implants, diagnostics, clinical treatments, and intervention methods. House researchers work with House Clinic physicians to integrate medicine and science through clinical and research trials.

House Ear Institute (HEI)
2100 West 3rd Street
Los Angeles, CA 90057
Phone:  (213) 483-4431
(in United States) (800) 388-8612
TDD (213) 484-2642
FAX (213) 483-8789

**International Hearing Society (IHS):** http://www.ihsinfo.org   IHS is the nonprofit, professional association that represents hearing instrument specialists in the United States, Canada, Japan, and several other countries. IHS advocates for and supports the highest standard of professional competency, business integrity, and excellence in serving the hearing impaired.

16880 Middlebelt Road, Suite 4
Livonia, MI 48154
(734) 522-7200

**John Tracy Clinic:** http://www.johntracyclinic.org   John Tracy Clinic provides, worldwide and without charge, parent-centered services to foster communication skills in young children with a hearing loss. The clinic also offers services to help the professional community understand how to work with deaf children. This site has a useful and informative FAQ page.

806 West Adams Boulevard
Los Angeles, CA 90007-2505
(213) 748-5481

**Laurent Clerc National Deaf Education Center:** http://clerc center.gallaudet.edu   Gallaudet University's Laurent Clerc National

Deaf Education Center shares the concerns of parents and professionals about the achievement of deaf and hard-of-hearing students in different learning environments across the country. The Clerc Center has been mandated by Congress to develop, evaluate, and disseminate innovative curricula, instructional techniques and strategies, and materials. The aim of the Clerc Center is to improve the quality of education for deaf and hard-of-hearing children and youth up to age 21.

> 800 Florida Avenue, NE
> Washington, DC 20002-3695
> (202) 651-5051

**The Listen Foundation:** http://www.listenfoundation.org The Listen Foundation has supported families who would otherwise not have access to the equipment and therapy that their children need in order to become listening, speaking adults, enabling them to reach their full potential as productive members of society.

> 6950 E. Belleview Avenue, Suite 203
> Englewood, CO 80111
> (303) 781-9440

**Listen-Up:** http://www.listen-up.org/index.htm Listen-Up provides information, answers, help, ideas, and resources related to hearing loss. Whether you're interested in auditory processing or buying a special alarm clock, the site will point you in the right direction. The Web master has dedicated years to gathering information and developing products geared to the special needs of hearing-impaired children and their families and professionals who serve them. He has firsthand experience dealing with hearing loss.

**The Marion Downs Hearing Center:** http://www.mariondowns.com The Marion Downs Hearing Center at the University of Colorado Hospital was created to honor the legacy of world-renowned audiologist, Marion Downs. The Center provides resources, education and research to support the needs of individuals who are deaf and hard of hearing, their families, the community and hearing health professionals.

> 1793 Quentin Street, Unit 2
> Aurora, CO 80045
> (720) 848 3042 (voice)
> TTY: (720) 848 2979

**MED-EL Corporation:**   http://www.medel.com/index_int.php
This cochlear implant manufacturer's Web site contains all kinds of
useful information not just about implants, but about the ear and
how it works.

2511 Old Cornwallis Road, Suite 100
Durham, NC 27713
(888) 633-3524

**My Baby's Hearing:** http://www.babyhearing.org   Boy's Town
National Research Hospital formed this Web site as an informative
resource for parents of babies with hearing loss, but it provides a
wealth of information for caregivers of infants with hearing loss as
well. Not only does this Web site teach about the ear and how it
works, it also describes different types of hearing loss a baby may
have and discusses causes for these hearing losses. It answers many
questions about the various styles of hearing aids and assistive
devices available for young children today. There is a small section
that discusses cochlear implants as an option for some babies with
hearing loss. This site teaches parents what type of testing to expect
for their child in future months and years. It explains in detail the
importance of the Universal Newborn Hearing Screening Program
and what it means if a child fails the screening. The Web site also
helps parents read and understand an audiogram. This is especially
important, as an audiogram will be used many times during future
hearing testing.

Boys Town National Research Hospital
555 N. 30th Street
Omaha, NE 68131
(402) 498-1438

**National Association of the Deaf:** http://www.nad.org   The
National Association of the Deaf (NAD), established in 1880, is
the oldest and largest constituency organization safeguarding
the accessibility and civil rights of 28 million deaf and hard–of–
hearing Americans in education, employment, health care, and
telecommunications.

8630 Fenton Street, Suite 820
Silver Spring, MD 20910-3819
(301) 587-1788

**National Centre for Audiology, Canada (NCA):** http://www
.uwo.ca/nca/   Canada's preeminent center of excellence in the
field of hearing health care, NCA houses Canada's largest educational and research programs in the field. NCA responsibilities
include continuing education and technical assistance for audiologists; research on hearing and hearing instruments; state-of-the-art
clinical services; consultation with government agencies, professional and consumer associations, and other agencies to improve
hearing health care services and public education about hearing
and hearing loss; and dissemination of knowledge about hearing
loss, its prevention, and treatment.

> University of Western Ontario
> Elborn College, Room 2262
> 1201 Western Road
> London, ON, Canada N6G 1H1
> (519) 661-3901

**National Center for Hearing Assessment and Management
(NCHAM):** http://www.infanthearing.org   The NCHAM site contains a wealth of information and resources concerning the many
dimensions of early hearing detection and intervention.

> Utah State University
> 2880 Old Main Hill
> Logan, UT 84322
> (435) 797-3584

**National Cued Speech Organization:** http://www.cuedspeech
.org   The National Cued Speech Association is a nonprofit membership organization founded in 1982 to promote and support the
effective use of Cued Speech. This organization raises awareness of
Cued Speech and its applications, provides educational services,
assists local affiliate chapters, establishes standards for Cued Speech,
and certifies Cued Speech instructors and transliterators.

> 5619 McLean Drive
> Bethesda, MD 20814-1021
> (800) 459-3529

**National Early Childhood Technical Assistance Center
(NECTAC):** http://www.nectac.org   The NECTAC Web site supports
the implementation of the early childhood provisions of the Indi-

viduals with Disabilities Education Improvement Act (IDEA). This technical assistance focuses on early childhood research, "best practices," and policy and legal issues. The mission of the Center is to strengthen service systems to ensure that children with disabilities up to age five (and their families) receive and benefit from high quality, culturally appropriate, and family-centered supports and services. Through the Web site the knowledge base of early intervention and early childhood special education is made available in a variety of formats.

NECTAC
517 South Greensboro Street
Carrboro, NC 27510
(919) 962-2001

**National Institute on Deafness and Other Communication Disorders (NIDCD):** http://www.nidcd.nih.gov   The NIDCD conducts research on disorders of human communication, including hearing, balance, smell, taste, voice, speech, and language. This site includes a nice interactive section for teachers and children.

31 Center Drive, MSC 2320
Bethesda, MD 20892-2320
(301) 496-7243

**Otikids:** http://www.otikids.com   Sponsored by hearing aid manufacturer Oticon, this Web site has lots of helpful information for parents and kids, including testimonials from children around the world who wear hearing aids and from their parents.

**Oral Deaf Education:** http://www.oraldeafed.org   This organization is dedicated to helping deaf children learn to talk. The new technology available today through modern hearing aids and cochlear implants provides access to sound that, with appropriate technology and instruction at Oral Deaf Education Schools, most deaf children can learn to talk.

**Parents of Deaf HH:** Parents of Deaf HH is a listserv of parents of deaf and hard-of-hearing children. This on-line support group is a useful tool for parents who have questions or need encouragement while raising their deaf children. E-mail: parentdeafhh@listserv.kent.edu

**Phonak:** http://www.phonak.com/   Link to the Phonak Web site to learn about its hearing aids. The Web site has a useful section devoted to pediatric hearing loss including a simulation of mild and moderate hearing loss (under the "Consumer" section).

4520 Weaver Parkway
Warrenville, IL 60555
(800) -679-4871

**Raising Deaf Kids:** http://raisingdeafkids.org   The Children's Hospital of Philadelphia formed this Web site as a resource for parents and caregivers of children who are hard of hearing or deaf. This Web site, which can also be viewed in Spanish, answers questions about hearing loss, gives excellent communication tips, and aids parents in making communication decisions. It also contains links to a number of resources (organizations, books, and Web sites) that may be useful to parents or caregivers.

3440 Market Street, 4th Floor
Behavioral Health Center
Philadelphia, PA 19104
(215) 590-7440

**SayWhatClub:** http://www.saywhatclub.com   The SayWhatClub is a non-profit, tax-exempt organization dedicated to enhancing interpersonal communication for people who are deaf, hard-of-hearing, or have a serious interest in hearing loss. Its goals include providing online space for deaf and hard-of-hearing people to share experiences, frustrations, and support; and educating participants and the public about all aspects of hearing loss.

**S.E.E. Center for the Advancement of Deaf Children:** http://www.seecenter.org/   The S.E.E. Center is a nonprofit organization that works with parents and educators of hard-of-hearing children. The center promotes early identification and intervention, as well as information about the sign language system, Signing Exact English, and workshops to train people to use it.

P.O. Box 1181
Los Alamitos, CA 90720
(562) 430-1467

**Siemens:** http://www.siemens-hearing.com This hearing aid manufacturer's Web site contains information about its products as well as a useful site about pediatric hearing loss.

153 E. 53rd Street
New York, NY 10022
(800) 743-6367

**Ski Hi Institute:** http://www.skihi.org/ The SKI-HI Institute is a group of parents and professionals whose goal is to enhance the lives of young children with special needs and their families. Many programs have been developed at the SKI-HI Institute for children who are deaf or hard of hearing, blind/visually impaired, deaf-blind, multi-disabled, or have any special needs.

6500 Old Main Hill
Logan, UT 84322-6500
(435) 797-5600

**Strategies for Teaching Children:** http://www.as.wvu.edu/~sci dis/hearing.html This Web site introduces strategies for teaching children with hearing impairments.

**VOICE for Hearing Impaired Children:** http://voicefordeafkids .com The mission of this organization is to ensure that all hearing-impaired children have the right to develop their ability to listen and speak and have access to services that will enable them to listen and speak. VOICE is based in Toronto, and assists in making effective decisions by providing information regarding the available choices and the ongoing support required for these choices. VOICE promotes parental choice regarding communicative approaches for deaf children with the auditory-verbal approach as the first option. The Web site also provides a forum for parents to discuss their individual concerns and gain support from one another.

161 Eglinton Avenue East, Suite 701
Toronto, ON, Canada M4P 1J5
(866) 779-5144

# INDEX